Stress Can't Always Be Avoided— but Your Attitude Can Make a Big Difference!

- Do you make mountains out of molehills?
- Do you know *how* to say no?
- Do you unconsciously pick the *worst* times to argue with your loved ones or your boss?
- Does the holiday rush destroy the fun for you?
- Do you know that weather can make you anxious, irritable, fatigued?
- Are you aware that lying can make you sick?
- Do you protect yourself from the jarring effects of loud noise?
- Do you eat the right foods and take the right vitamins to alleviate stress?

Good news! Now you *can* change stress-producing attitudes that make you too fearful, vulnerable, demanding, pessimistic or judgmental. You *can* reduce stress, use your energy more productively, and head toward a happier, more positive, more healthful life with . . .

CONQUERING STRESS

Books from The NATIONAL ENQUIRER

Conquering Stress
Famous Disasters
Living with Arthritis
UFO Report

Published by POCKET BOOKS

NATIONAL ENQUIRER

ENQUIRER

CONQUERING
STRESS

PUBLISHED BY POCKET BOOKS NEW YORK

Material in this book is based on articles previously published in The NATIONAL ENQUIRER.

The Baylor College of Medicine stress plan was extracted from Baylor College of Medicine's WE CARE FOR YOU health promotion series.

Another *Original* publication of POCKET BOOKS

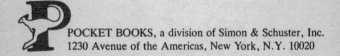

POCKET BOOKS, a division of Simon & Schuster, Inc.
1230 Avenue of the Americas, New York, N.Y. 10020

ISBN: 0-671-52839-4

First Pocket Books printing May, 1985

10 9 8 7 6 5 4 3 2 1

Contents

CONQUERING STRESS

Introduction

LIFE CAN BE ONE LONG TENSION HEADACHE. JOB pressures, family conflicts, money worries, world crises, health problems, overcrowding and the deafening roar of the world in motion, day after day, can make living—just the simple act of getting through life—an overwhelming chore. We all know what it is like to have kids who fight all the time or grocery bills that keep ringing up higher on the cash register each month. Everyone has had a boss yell at him or a husband who comes home and sits sullenly in front of the TV set without saying a word. Sometimes the hours just don't stretch far enough for all the things we need to get done.

In the end, whatever the specifics of our troubles, we are all suffering from the same problem—STRESS. The stress of fights and arguments. The stress of buying a new house, changing jobs, getting married, taking a test, starting a diet, beginning an exercise program, having a dinner party. Bad experiences or good, each and every event in our lives brings with it the stress of coping with what is happening. It can be a new arrival, such as a baby, which normally fills us with joy. But a baby also brings new strains to a marriage—too little sleep and unexpected expenses. Along with the wonders and joys of parenthood come the worries about whether you will be a good parent.

Take Mary and Robert L., a young married couple who, for seven years, have prided themselves on the "workability" of their relationship. They met in high school, married five months after graduating and both eventually found jobs. Mary is a secretary for a local life insurance company, likes her boss and fellow workers and sees the possibility of one day becoming a sales representative for the company.

Robert is an assistant manager at a trucking firm. He travels forty miles every day to get to his plant and has to work long hours two to three days a week. He likes his job, but realizes that he has probably gotten as far as he is going to with the company. But there aren't a lot of job opportunities around and Robert hasn't felt the need to actively search for a new position.

Mary and Robert have spent most of the past seven years fixing up a small one-bedroom house. It gives them a chance to be together and is a constructive way for them to spend their time in the evening and on weekends. Their marriage has been a good one—quiet, but fulfilling. They seldom argue—because they share the same goals. The fact that Mary works has allowed them to build a small nest egg of savings and the future looks rosy. Or does it?

SCENE I: Mary and Robert have finished dinner. It's Friday night and they are both relaxing after the long work week.

MARY: I've been thinking about having a baby. I started thinking about it the other day when Judy came into the office to visit with her six-month-old son.

ROBERT: But you're the one who didn't want to start a family yet. You always said there was plenty of time. Why do you want to jump into all this now?

MARY: I don't call wanting to have a child after seven years "jumping into" anything. In fact, I'd call it dragging your heels.

ROBERT: You mean you wanted to have a baby all along, and it's my fault we haven't had one! You know, your timing is incredible! Here I am looking for a new job and you want to have a baby. What are we going to live on? Have you thought of that?

MARY: What do you mean "looking for a new job"? I wasn't counting on your quitting your job the minute I said I wanted to have a child. Are you trying to punish me for wanting to be a mother?

ROBERT: I'm not trying to do anything. Here you are presenting me with one of the most important decisions we'll ever make, and you have already made up your mind. I haven't even been consulted and I'm supposed to be the father of this baby. Count me out.

Stress! Mary and Robert have just uncovered enough stress-inducing, tension-causing, anxiety-ridden issues to last a year. And they have done it in a way that is bound to result in disaster. Both of them are to blame. This scene could have been avoided.

First, Mary picks the end of the week, when they are both tired, to bring up a subject which is critical to both their lives and about which she appears to have already made a decision. In addition, Mary is all set for a battle, which is why she takes the role of the wounded victim of Robert's "punishment." She makes Robert into a bully, when, in fact, Mary's trying to bully Robert into going along with her wishes. If Mary had really been listening to Robert over the past months, she would have picked up on the signals he was giving her about wanting to find a new job.

Robert is hardly blameless in all this. He assumes that Mary's desire to have a baby is meant as a slap in the face. Just as Mary didn't pick up on Robert's job dissatisfaction, he has not paid attention to her hints about becoming a mother. And Robert's announcement that he is job hunting is just a ploy to focus the conversation back on him and away from the actual question of starting a family.

So, Mary and Robert share the blame. So what? The point is that there is stress and then there is STRESS! Some stress is unavoidable, but other types of stress are unnecessary. All of us can try to change ourselves and our habits so that we don't create even more stress in our lives. After all, there is a breaking point in each of us. There is a time when we just CAN'T TAKE ANY MORE!!!! Aren't there enough sources of anxiety and tension in the world that we cannot control? Do we have to add to it by being selfish or thoughtless or pigheaded? No. We can choose to create stress or choose to reduce it. We can change our habits, if we try to and if we have some guidance. That is what this book is all about. It will tell you how to handle daily stresses before they make you crazy. It will tell you about programs and exercises that can reduce the stress you feel. It will even tell you whether you are suffering from too little or too much stress. And it will show you what can happen if you continue to ignore the toll stress is taking on you, your life and your family.

Let's get back to Mary and Robert. We have seen

what they did wrong. Now let's see whether they can undo the damage they have caused.

SCENE II: It is Saturday morning. Robert slept on the couch all night and Mary locked the door to her bedroom and cried for hours. Both are angry and hurt. Both feel that they were treated unfairly. They meet in the kitchen, where Robert has just finished making the coffee.

ROBERT: I had a dream last night that we sold the house and moved to Jacksonville. I got a job at a lumberyard and you had twins. It was pretty rough at first, because we didn't have much money and taking care of the twins all day wore you out.

MARY: Did I cry all the time and scream at the kids?

ROBERT: Nope.

MARY: Did we fight a lot?

ROBERT: Nope.

MARY: Did I listen to you when you tried to tell me what was wrong at work?

ROBERT: Yep. We talked about the options—what we could afford to do financially and what I really wanted from my job.

MARY: Hey! I think I was having the same dream. I remember talking with you about having a baby while we were still young enough. We spent months planning the expenses and how we would manage together. I remember slowing down, not demanding instant motherhood, but figuring out whether our marriage was strong enough to include children. Was that the dream you had?

ROBERT: Sounds like it to me.

* * *

The resolution to Mary and Robert's problems may seem a little too slick to be real. But it is important to remember the power of compromise. There are times when you should act on impulse and times when two heads are better than one. With thought and caring and discipline, you can reduce the stress of your life. Whether you are dealing with your boss, your children, your friends or strangers; traffic jams, supermarket lines, doctors' offices or family picnics—there is the stress inherent in the situation and the stress you bring with you as you deal with it. You *do* have control over your life. It may take a little more effort and time, but you can determine whether your stress is a burden you can bear or a force that carries you along with it to an unknown destination.

CHAPTER I

Stress Awareness

STRESS. THERE IS NO WAY TO AVOID IT. IT CAN'T BE cured by medicine, surgery, transplants or black magic. But you can live with stress, use it to your advantage and come to appreciate it once you learn how to.

Those of us who recognize the symptoms of stress usually look for an obvious cause—illness, the death of a loved one or family and financial problems. Yet, surprisingly enough, some of the best things in life— some of the rewards we hope for and work for—can bring the greatest stress to our lives. If you win the lottery or inherit money from a rich uncle, you suddenly discover that everyone wants to help you spend your money. Relatives and lawyers and get-rich-quick schemers come out of the woodwork. And you find you have traded your worries about paying the rent for worries about how dramatically to change your lifestyle without losing the values that are most important to you.

Or suppose you suddenly get the supervisory position you have slaved toward over the years. All your hard work has paid off and money problems are a thing of the past. And, just as suddenly, you start thinking you can't handle this new job. The hours you are expected to spend at the office are putting a terrific strain on your family life. What if you fail? What if you get fired? Anxiety can turn this rich reward into a nightmare.

It doesn't seem fair. We expect to worry about the bad things, but nobody told us the good things in life could have the same negative impact. Here is where your understanding of stress and your attitude toward it are vital.

If you don't learn how to control stress, stress will control you. Given all the aspects of life you cannot control—like fires and recessions and accidents—don't you want to take advantage of advice that can put you in the driver's seat for a change? It is your decision.

How to Know
If You're Suffering from Stress

It is estimated that 60 to 70 percent of the people who go to see a doctor suffer from symptoms of stress, rather than symptoms of a particular illness. Stomach disorders, aching backs, sleeping problems, loss of appetite, headaches, depression and dozens more symptoms can be related to stress. Of course, they can also indicate serious illness, so you should always let your doctor decide whether you have a specific disease.

What are the symptoms? Dr. Hans Selye, who is considered to be the "father" of stress research, provides an extensive list of "self-observable" signs of stress in his famous book, *The Stress of Life*. These are the indications we can see for ourselves, if we know what to look for. Here is Dr. Selye's list:

1. General irritability, hyperexcitation or depression

2. Pounding of the heart
3. Dryness of the throat or mouth
4. Impulsive behavior, emotional instability
5. The overpowering urge to cry or run and hide
6. Inability to concentrate
7. Feelings of unreality, weakness or dizziness
8. Predeliction (inclination) to become fatigued
9. "Floating anxiety" (fear of something, but not any one particular thing)
10. Emotional tension and alertness, feeling of being "keyed up"
11. Trembling, nervous tics
12. Tendency to be easily startled
13. High-pitched, nervous laughter
14. Stuttering and speech difficulties
15. Bruxism, or grinding of the teeth
16. Insomnia (the inability to sleep)
17. Hypermotility (moving around randomly, without a specific reason)
18. Sweating
19. The frequent need to urinate
20. Diarrhea, indigestion, queasiness in the stomach and sometimes even vomiting
21. Migraine headaches
22. Premenstrual tension or missed menstrual cycles
23. Pain in the neck and lower back
24. Loss of or excessive appetite
25. Increased smoking
26. Increased use of legally prescribed drugs, such as tranquilizers or amphetamines
27. Alcohol and drug addiction
28. Nightmares
29. Neurotic behavior
30. Psychoses
31. Accident proneness

* * *

Now, just because you do not have all, or even a majority of these "symptoms," does not mean you aren't under a great deal of stress. Each person reacts differently and has his own areas of weakness. Some people become depressed, lose their appetite, drink too much and sleep poorly when they are exposed to more stress than they can handle. Others become very aggressive, pace the floor for hours, are keyed up and laugh almost hysterically for no real reason. This list simply provides warning signals. They can help you to recognize that you have a problem. This is the first step. The next step is to quantify the problem—is it a major problem or a minor one?

Simple Tests to Find Your Stress Level

How much stress are you under? Dr. Selye's list of stress signs is comprehensive, but it doesn't give us a sense, necessarily, of just how much stress we are suffering from. There are a multitude of stress tests that use a scoring system to appoint individual values to your response to stress.

Dr. John Farquhar, director of the heart disease prevention program at Stanford University School of Medicine in California, outlines one stress test in his book, *The American Way of Life Need Not Be Hazardous to Your Health.* He uses it as part of a self-help antistress plan he developed along with other authorities in the Stanford program.

The first step is to answer each question by using one of the following three responses: often, a few times a week, rarely.

1. I feel tense, anxious or have nervous indigestion.   Answer: _____

2. People at work/home arouse my tension.   Answer: _____

3. I eat/drink/smoke in response to tension.   Answer: _____

4. I have tension or migraine headaches, pain in neck or shoulders or insomnia.   Answer: _____

5. I can't turn off my thoughts at night or on the weekends long enough to feel relaxed the next day.   Answer: _____

6. I find it difficult to concentrate on what I'm doing because of worrying about other things.   Answer: _____

7. I take tranquilizers (or other drugs) to relax.   Answer: _____

8. I have a difficult time finding enough time to relax.   Answer: _____

ANSWER THE FOLLOWING QUESTIONS EITHER YES OR NO

9. Once I find the time, it's hard for me to relax.   Answer: _____

10. My workday is made
    up of many deadlines.   Answer: _____

It is easy to score yourself on this test. According to your response, put the following numbers right next to each answer. When you have all the numbers filled in, add them up and compare your score to the ones below.

> Often = 2 points
> A few times a week and Yes = 1 point
> Rarely and No = 0 points

If you scored 14–18 points, you are considerably above average in stress; 10–13 points means you are above average; 6–9 points are average; 3–5 points means you're below average; and 0–2 equals well below average.

No matter how you scored, you can benefit from learning stress management techniques. And, if you scored in the "above average" or "considerably above average" range, Dr. Farquhar suggests that you start a program for coping with stress, either by consulting your doctor or by learning how to relax.

There are other signs of stress that may not be obvious at all. You might want to add them to Dr. Selye's list of thirty-one symptoms.

Another Stanford University expert, Dr. Alejandro Martinez, who teaches stress management techniques, adds five other telltale and "hidden" signs of stress. He includes catching colds or the flu frequently and having the symptoms hang on longer than normal; experiencing muscle tension and spasms, and other aches and pains that seem to have no physical cause; starting to feel futile and inadequate, and losing interest in things that used to concern you; increasing strain in your relations with friends and loved ones, and frequent shows of temper; and worrying a lot about what is wrong with you.

Taken individually, each of these conditions may be a symptom of some other physical or emotional problem. But, if you suffer from a majority of them—in addition to other signs of emotional and physical strain—you are probably a victim of *hidden stress,* says Dr. Martinez.

Hidden stress is one danger. *Stress addiction* is another. It may be hard to imagine, but there are people who seem to thrive on tension. They love deadlines, seemingly impossible tasks, taking unnecessary risks, last-minute crises.

Dr. Herbert Hoffman, a psychologist and director of the Hillside Psychological Guidance Center in Queens Village, New York, has developed a quiz to determine whether you are a stress addict. Some people are actually hooked on stress and go out of their way to find crisis situations. While getting involved in stressful situations can be exhilarating, it can also be hazardous to your health.

To find out if you're addicted to stress, answer each of the following questions.

1. Do you often find yourself working like crazy to meet deadlines? (A) Yes. (B) No.

2. If you had to attend an important meeting in an unfamiliar part of town, would you get careful directions for reaching your destination before leaving? (A) Yes. (B) No.

3. Do you have a reputation for being (A) early or (B) late for appointments?

4. Some people stop to get gas only when the fuel gauge is hovering on empty. Within the last six months, have you (A) done this often or (B) not done this more than once or twice?

5. Do you usually file tax returns, pay bills, return library books, get license plates or renew your driver's license (A) at the very last minute or (B) well ahead of time?

6. Do you make it a habit to pet strange dogs? (A) Yes. (B) No.

7. Do you think you are at your best when there's a crisis? (A) Yes. (B) No.

8. Within the last six months, have you gone shopping only to find that you have left your wallet, checkbook and your credit cards at home? (A) Yes. (B) No.

9. When taking children to an amusement park, would you prefer to take them on (A) the roller coaster or (B) the merry-go-round?

SCORING: Assign yourself the correct number of points for each question by following this chart. Then total your score.

Question 1: (A) 1 point	(B) 0 points	
Question 2: (A) 0	(B) 1	
Question 3: (A) 0	(B) 1	
Question 4: (A) 1	(B) 0	
Question 5: (A) 1	(B) 0	
Question 6: (A) 1	(B) 0	
Question 7: (A) 1	(B) 0	
Question 8: (A) 1	(B) 0	
Question 9: (A) 1	(B) 0	

Dr. Hoffman's analysis of the scoring system is interesting. Low scores (0 to 3) show that you are in virtually no danger of being a stress addict. "If anything, you are more apt to be suffering from boredom," Dr. Hoffman says, "for you tend to play it safe on most occasions." The remedy? Try something new. "If life at times appears to be unbearably dull and routine, you could benefit by exposing yourself to a few novel experiences. You need not do anything dangerous to make your life more exciting. Resolve to be more open to new friendships, explore new interests and investigate the possibility that you have been squelching your latent talents and abilities by your dedication to living cautiously."

A middle range score (4 to 6) shows that you "maintain a healthy balance between risk taking and prudent caution, and thus are not likely to become a stress addict," Dr. Hoffman advises. "You undoubtedly become involved in stressful situations from time to time, but it is unlikely you have sought them out. You rarely exceed your own levels of stress endurance, and you minimize the effects of stress on your life by accepting your own limitations."

A high score (7 to 9) is an important warning signal that "you are either a true stress addict or perilously close to becoming one," Dr. Hoffman warns. "It would be wise for you to begin at once to take steps to alter this dangerous, self-destructive behavior pattern and wean yourself from the thrill of living at so high a level of speed and intensity."

We will discuss in a later chapter the advice Dr. Hoffman and others offer on how to live life with less stress.

Do You Suffer from Stress Deficiency?

As we have just seen, too little stress can lead to a boring life. It can also be just as destructive as too much stress, according to some experts. And the problem is more widespread than you might think. Nearly 20 million people suffer from stress deficiency.

Do you watch a lot of TV lately? Have you lost

interest in current affairs or lost touch with local issues? Are you having difficulty getting up in the morning? Does each day seem just like the day before? Are you vaguely aware of a feeling that life isn't much fun, even though things are going pretty smoothly? If you answered "yes" to three or more of these questions, you may be a victim of too little stress, according to two leading mental-health experts.

Dr. Hoffman, whom we have already met as the stress addict analyst, says stress deficiency is a "major, usually unrecognized problem, far more common than most people suspect." Dr. James A. Giannini, associate professor of psychiatry at Northeastern Ohio College of Medicine in Youngstown agrees, adding that "most people are all too familiar with stress overload. They become alarmed when recurrent problems, complicated by anxiety, exhaustion, strain and tension, bring them close to the breaking point. But few individuals understand that when you get up each day feeling 'Ho-hum, I know exactly what's going to happen today—nothing,' you're under-stressed and in as much trouble as when you wake up frantic with all you have to do."

Dr. Giannini says the dominant signs are headaches, acting in a snappy manner, ignoring the people around you, not completing your work, not being able to concentrate on recreational reading, a "nothing matters" attitude and a general retreat from life.

Dr. Hoffman says the profile of a stress deficient person is "an over-achiever, over-doer, over-striver" who suddenly decides he can't do it anymore. He feels that he has to dramatically reduce his burden of stress and overreacts by going from too much to too little stress. "He mentally gives up," Dr. Hoffman explains. "If formerly superambitious, he may retreat to an 'along-for-the-ride' work attitude; if once 'gung-ho' to make his mark, he may voluntarily take a lower-level job. He seems to adopt a 'what's-the-use' approach to life, essentially retreating from the very activeness he once found so enjoyable."

Take the case of Mike, who graduated from high school and immediately got two jobs. One was as a night janitor in a printing firm. The other was more to Mike's liking because of the nature of the business. He was assistant manager of a local steak house. Mike liked the responsibility, talking with the customers, even handling complaints. He could see himself with his own restaurant one day, buying a franchise in a large chain of steak houses.

After two years of working 75-hour weeks, Mike decided it was time to devote all of his energy to the restaurant business. He was up for a promotion to manager, which would require more of his time and paid well enough for him to drop his second job.

Then two months after Mike got the promotion to manager, he was asked to take on the added responsibility of starting up another steak house on the other side of town. This meant longer hours once again and constant running back and forth between the two places. Mike's customers started noticing that he never had time for them, and when they greeted him he barely acknowledged their hellos. Two waitresses quit on the same day, after Mike accused them of goofing off on the job. Suppliers started complaining that their bills were not being paid on time, and Mike began to take longer and longer lunch hours—sometimes disappearing for the whole afternoon. His appearance became sloppy, and he often forgot to wear a jacket and tie to work. Finally, Mike's boss called him up to find out if anything was wrong, and Mike, in a fury over being "cross-examined," quit. Mike's boss was shocked. How was it possible that his star employee, the one he used to boast about all over town, had changed so completely?

Mike was suffering from stress deficiency. If Dr. Hoffman's theory is to be applied here, Mike simply gave up after a period of "stress-overload." Stress-deficient people withdraw into themselves. They become self-centered. "Their conversation can be a dead giveaway to what's happening," Dr. Hoffman says. "They'll talk about their health, their bowel movements, how well or how poorly they slept last night, little aches and pains and whether it is too hot or too cold, too dry or too rainy for them to go outside."

And you do not have to be actively employed in a high-pressure job to come up against the "stress-deficiency" problem. Retired executives, teachers, "empty nest" mothers and anyone who once lived a pressure-filled life may end up going to the other extreme of giving up or retreating from life.

Stress deficiency can be very dangerous. Dr. Giannini found that this condition often brings with it a desire to "break out of the blahs" by doing something life threatening. One patient took up skydiving, and each time he jumped he kept delaying opening the parachute. Others have taken up gambling, speeding, driving on the wrong side of the road or shoplifting. Men sometimes start flirtations in the office or become argumentative with their bosses.

Stress as a Medical Problem

Many, perhaps most, experts today believe that stress is the *process of coping* with the events in life, not the events themselves. For instance, if you have saved some money and decide to go shopping for a dress, this event is not stressful in itself. You see something you like, it fits you and the occasions for which you will need it and you buy it. It is a happy situation with very little stress attached to it. It is gratifying to find what you want, to purchase it and to be able to afford it.

However, if, while you go through this activity of getting a new dress, you think "I should spend this money on the children's clothes, not mine," or you say to yourself, "I'm too fat . . . I should lose some weight before I get a new dress . . . and besides, I never go anywhere; what do I need a new dress for?" then you are creating stress that is not inherent in the act of buying a dress. The dress does not contain the elements of stress, but your impression of what the dress represents—wasted money, figure flaws, unfulfilled desires—brings stress to it.

On the other hand, "father stress" himself, Dr. Hans Selye, says that stress cannot be avoided no matter what we do: "There is a demand on the body to provide the energy to maintain life and to deal with changing influences outside ourselves. Even asleep we are under some stress, as our vital organs continue to function and the brain dreams. Complete freedom from stress is death."

Whichever theory you find more compelling, certain facts about the physical effects of stress are widely agreed upon. Your body goes through many processes during moments of stress. Whether it is "good" stress, like getting praise for your work, or "bad" stress, such as getting a cold or fighting with your wife, your body reacts in the same way. Hormones and other chemicals are released into the bloodstream, blood pressure fluctuates and the brain is stimulated. The skin reacts by growing cold or hot and sweating. The immune system, which is an internal defense system for fighting infection, is activated. It is a reminder of how incredibly intricate and complicated the body is. We each have a whole-body reaction system that is activated by stress.

Now let's take a look at some of the *adverse* "side effects" of stress:

Stress is the most widespread medical problem in America today. It's a major contributing factor in 100 percent of diseases. No one is immune.

> —*Dr. Alfred Coodley, psychiatrist,*
> *University of Southern California*
> *Medical School*

Stress upsets the stomach and brings on ulcers, stress boosts blood pressure, leading to strokes and heart attacks. Stress can turn you into an alcoholic or a dope addict—a trading of one evil for another which is just as deadly.

> —*Dr. Robert L. Woolfolk and*
> *Dr. Frank C. Richardson,*
> *psychologists, and coauthors of*
> Stress, Sanity and Survival

Many heart-related deaths occur in apparently healthy people with no evidence of heart disease or artery blockage. . . . There must be an additional factor in sudden cardiac deaths—and that factor is stress.

> —*Dr. James Skinner, neurophysiologist,*
> *Baylor College of Medicine*

When we're faced with stressful situations, our bodies "gear up" to meet the challenge. Some scientists say that we react just as our primitive ancestors did when faced with wild animals or other life-threatening conditions—with a "fight-or-flight" response. When the brain sounds the "danger" signal, an entire set of physical responses takes place—including an increase in the heart rate, so that more blood can be pumped into the skeletal muscles.

This kind of "battle alert" may have helped our ancestors deal with the dangers they faced, and it can be useful still for soldiers going into battle. But experts say it isn't very useful for solving the complex problems of modern life.

For example, a tough boss is not the same kind of problem as a saber-toothed tiger, and, if you respond to criticism from your boss with "fight-or-flight" behavior, you're probably going to find yourself out of a job. If you have a "fight" reaction to this same employer and simply choke back your anger and frustration, you may keep your job—but you may develop chronic and life-shortening health problems. When we are stressed too severely and/or too long, we can develop what experts call "stress sickness."

Stress can knock out your immune system. Stress can make you sick by wreaking havoc on your immune system, allowing disease to strike much more easily. "Stress causes the white blood cells of the immune system to be greatly altered, and this allows sickness to set in," says Dr. Robert S. Brown, clinical associate professor of psychiatry and behavioral medicine at the University of Virginia. "What happens is this: in case of danger or threat, our bodies pour out hormones, which give us additional strength, so we can fight or run away. This was very useful in primitive times, but today it often works against us. In the civilized world, we can't fight or run away from our problems. So the extra energy isn't used. Instead, it remains in the body, harming us by weakening our immune system."

Dr. Brown says that stress-triggered disease usually attacks whatever weak spot already exists. In smokers, for example, the attack would take place in the lungs.

Stress and atherosclerosis. If your heart pounds and adrenaline pumps through your veins during stressful situations, chances are you're a candidate for atherosclerosis, or hardening of the arteries. And you're twice as likely to develop the potentially fatal disease if you're a leader, rather than a follower, a fascinating study revealed.

Researchers at the Bowman Gray Medical School in Winston-Salem, North Carolina, conducted a twenty-one-month-long study on thirty macaque monkeys—animals physically similar to humans. Fifteen of the monkeys were kept under stress and the other fifteen in nonstressful situations. At the end of the study, the researchers found that dominant monkeys under stress tended to have faster heartbeats. Furthermore, these same monkeys had nearly twice the amount of arteriosclerosis than the others.

The researchers couldn't explain these differences by what are commonly considered the traditional risk factors for atherosclerosis—blood pressure, cholesterol and blood constituents, said Dr. Jay R. Kaplan, Ph.D., who conducted the study with two colleagues. Instead, they linked the atherosclerosis to hormones called *catecholamines,* which are secreted at high levels by the body under stress, and which adversely affect the blood and blood vessels.

Dr. Stephen Manuck, one of Dr. Kaplan's collaborators in the study, said the chances were excellent that the same stress results apply to humans. Dr. Manuck, a clinical psychologist and a psychophysiologist, is an expert on stress and its effects on the cardiovascular system. "Our study is important because it's pointing to the same sorts of things in humans," he explained. "If you take a dominant personality human and put him in a stressful environment, he is more apt to react with high blood pressure and a pounding heart . . . and he is more apt to suffer damage to his arteries over the long term."

Dr. William Castelli, the director of the famous Framingham (Massachusetts) Heart Study, said "This is a very exciting study. We know that Type A males and females run about twice the heart attack rate as Type Bs. We know that stress seems to be an important risk factor. And now here's an experimental model where this happens in animals.

"That's now proving the scientific consistency, saying that, not only does it exist in epidemiological studies, but, when you go into animals and make a model, it works in the model in exactly the same ratio as it does with humans.

"That's very impressive. And I think it's a lesson for all of us: we ought to start looking for that other drummer and try to calm down!"

Are You a "Type A" Personality?

Take a long, honest look at yourself. Are you a competitive, impatient person? Do you walk and eat quickly? Do you finish other people's sentences? Do you hate to wait in line? Do you prefer talking to listening?

Does your life center around achievements? Do you like to do two things at once? Do you schedule too much in too little time? Are you always rushing? If you take time to relax, do you feel guilty?

These are some of the characteristics of a Type A personality, as described by cardiologists Dr. Meyer Friedman and Dr. Ray H. Rosenman in *Type A Behavior and Your Heart*.

The doctors studied three thousand men over an eight-year period to determine the effects, if any, that being a Type A personality might have on a person's health. Type As were found to be twice as likely to get heart disease as the more relaxed Type Bs.

Mental stress could be a killer. The "killing factor" in sudden cardiac deaths may be mental stress—and this could explain why, for example, voodoo curses can kill.

"Many heart-related deaths occur in apparently healthy people with no evidence of heart disease or artery blockage," observes Dr. James Skinner of Baylor College of Medicine. On the other hand, he points out that millions of people with heart disease go on living.

"There must be an additional factor in sudden cardiac deaths—and that factor is stress," says Dr. Skinner, a specialist in the makeup of the nervous system. He suggests that deaths from voodoo curses provide evidence that the mind, or nervous system, can trigger a heart attack.

Dr. Skinner cites the pioneering studies of famed physiologist Walter Cannon: "In the 1930s, Cannon traveled the world, studying voodoo-curse deaths in primitive cultures. He became convinced that people in the prime of health could die if they believed they were under a voodoo hex. His conclusion was that mental stress was sufficient to cause their deaths."

Dr. Skinner says that three separate present-day studies have found that 15 percent of the people who drop dead from so-called heart attacks do not suffer any heart-related disease. "We know," he says, "that these people who are dying suddenly are actually dying from ventricular fibrillation (heart spasms). Our research and that of others suggests that a brain factor alone can be quite sufficient to bring on ventricular fibrillation. We can stimulate certain parts of the brain electrically and cause this to happen (in laboratory animals)." Dr. Skinner believes that the same effect could be produced in humans by stress.

These are just a few examples of how stress can take a toll on our bodies. Remember that we are each equipped with the mechanisms and systems for coping with stress. Our bodies can endure stress. The point is not to let stress get so out of control. Stomach ulcers, digestion problems, headaches, heart attacks and—some doctors believe—even cancer can all result from stress overload. And marital problems, anger, frustration, depression, job troubles, eating problems and endless other conditions can come from our inability to deal with stress effectively or our ignorance of how we should cope with stress.

The rest of this book will deal with common stresses and how to manage them. There are ideas on how to change your attitudes and habits; exercises and total programs to help you get through the stress of life without succumbing to it. There are ways you can learn to look at your life to determine what things bother you most and what to do about them. You are the only one who can decide whether you want to change. It is a challenge that can improve your life—and perhaps save it.

CHAPTER II

Managing Stress— It's a Question of Attitude

THE TURNING POINT IN DEALING WITH STRESS STARTS with your attitude. Whether you believe that stress is totally dependent on outside influences and events, or you believe that stress is a result of how you perceive and react to the pressures of living, the critical factor is you. You are the one who has to live with the pressure and strain of everyday existence. And you alone can determine the quality of your life.

Seven Steps to Overcoming Stress

The following seven steps cover a wide range of harmful and helpful attitudes toward stress. The emphasis is on changing our perceptions of people, situations and events in life which bring us more stress than they have to.

STEP 1: CONQUER "AWFULIZING"

List all the sources of stress in your life and give them a score of 10. Then write down the word "me" and give it a score of 90. Your total is 100 percent and you have just learned that 90 percent of the trouble is YOU. Dr. Jay Segal, director of Temple University's Stress Research and Biofeedback Laboratory, is convinced that 90 percent of stress is caused by our attitudes, personality traits and habits of "awfulizing" situations. To reduce this stress Dr. Segal says you must conquer five attitudes:

- fear
- vulnerability
- being too demanding
- being too judgmental
- being so pessimistic that you make any bad situation an awful one.

All of us are guilty at one time or another of these attitudes.

Here are several examples demonstrating the five attitudes. They are followed by Dr. Segal's explanation of how they cause most stress—and what you can do to change these attitudes:

FEAR. "You never get rid of a fear unless you face it," he says. Identify the source of your fear. Visualize yourself calm and confident, dealing with your life without fear. Then try to conquer your fear gradually.

For example, if you're afraid of dogs, don't force yourself to fondle a Doberman pinscher. Instead, begin by petting a puppy. "Work your way out of your fear step by step," Dr. Segal advises.

TOO DEMANDING. This is the most common stress-producing trait. We demand things of other people and of ourselves. And the more our demands go unmet or unsatisfied, the more stress we suffer.

Carolyn is a good example of a highly demanding, highly stressed personality. A perfectionist by nature, she felt there was a "right" way to do everything—and, of course, this was her way. By constantly imposing her values and her standards on people around her—family, friends and coworkers—Carolyn found herself constantly frustrated and stressed when other people did not meet her demands.

Worst of all, she suffered tremendously on the occasions when she herself could not meet her own high standards—when she was feeling sick or tired or simply not up to doing everything "perfectly."

"Take time to reappraise the demands you're making," Dr. Segal suggests. "Then eliminate those that are unnecessary or lead to frustration because they're not being met."

VULNERABILITY. A vulnerable person is a worrier. He blames his problems on outside forces.

After a messy divorce that followed her discovery that her husband was having an affair with his secretary, Lisa became more vulnerable than ever in her relationships with the opposite sex.

No sooner does she get involved with a new man than she begins to look for signs that he is doing something hurtful. If a week goes by without a phone call, Lisa concludes that the man has lost interest in her. Without taking the time to find out if he is busy or preoccupied, Lisa is apt to generate a confrontation in which she accuses her boyfriend of not caring, of leading her on—or of cheating on her. If the relationship breaks up, Lisa decides that she was right and that the man was a bad person—without realizing that often it's her own attitude that brings about the very thing she's afraid will happen.

"Instead of always seeing yourself as a victim, see if it's not your own values and beliefs that contribute to your anxiety," Dr. Segal advises. "Don't accept bad situations. Take control."

TOO PESSIMISTIC. For example, you miss a bus for work and you immediately tell yourself you're going to be fired. People who think like this are "terminal pessimists," Dr. Segal says.

To eliminate this stress-maker, he advises: "Think back to all the things you worried about that never happened. Once you realize that most worries are groundless, you'll worry less and less."

In addition, you can write down the things that would really be awful in your life. Then, when some minor inconvenience occurs, compare it with the situations that are truly awful.

TOO JUDGMENTAL. This is judging a person by only one trait, usually a fault. Dr. Segal notes that by constantly finding fault you can become a person with a chip-on-the-shoulder attitude. This will lead to more inner stress.

STEP 2: COUNT STRESS AS A "BLESSING"

Do you ever remember having a string of bad luck and hearing someone—your grandmother maybe—say "Count your blessings, dear." Well, Dr. Robert Weinberger, a Houston psychologist, calls stress a blessing in disguise "as long as you recognize it for what it is—a sign that something is bothering you."

For example, let's say you've always enjoyed your job—up until the time your company hired a new supervisor who constantly seems to be picking on you. Now you're tense and irritable on the job; your stomach knots up in the morning and you're anxious all day long. These symptoms are a signal that there's a problem in your life that needs solving.

You may solve the problem by talking to the supervisor and trying to arrive at an understanding. If that doesn't bring about a great improvement, you may have to work on it further in your own head, for example, by saying to yourself: "This person has an abrasive personality. He (or she) may be insecure in this new job and taking that out on me. That's no reason to make myself miserable and allow my performance to suffer."

STEP 3: DEVELOP A STRESS-HARDY PERSONALITY

Once you get over the idea that stress is always to be avoided, you can learn to meet it head on and make it work for you.

"No one can consistently refuse to face problems, run away from difficulties, duck the hard decisions, ignore traumatic changes or take the 'easy way out,'" says Dr. Suzanne Kobasa, assistant professor of psychology at the University of Chicago. "Life is never that smooth or that simple."

And, once you accept these ideas, you can turn stress to your advantage, according to Dr. Kobasa and Dr. Salvatore B. Maddi, of the University of Chicago. Together, they studied 837 executives and found that some were "stress victims," while others were "hardy executives," people who actually thrived on stress. What was the difference?

"Despite all the warnings that stress is a real killer," Dr. Maddi explains, "our research shows that to avoid becoming a stress victim, you need only learn to take advantage of stress.

"We have found that there are psychological qualities that can inoculate an individual and make him resistant to stress." In his stress studies Dr. Maddi found that having a hardy personality can decrease by 50 percent the chance of illness due to stress.

Here is how you can develop a hardy personality and turn stress to your advantage:

● *Develop a desire to grapple with problems, instead of trying to run away from them.* "Each of us faces unexpected difficulties, disappointments, minor or major setbacks almost daily," says Dr. Kobasa. "When we shrink from those experiences, we eventually develop a sense of helplessness and hopelessness, which often leads to some sort of breakdown.

"But if you tell yourself: 'Here is a chance for me to take charge,' it gets your adrenaline going. You begin to feel that you control life, instead of it controlling you. Fears vanish, and you are stronger and healthier for the experience, whatever the outcome."

● *Welcome change.* "All of us are faced with changes in life," explains Dr. Maddi. "Since change is inevitable, we must learn to welcome it. Our 'hardy executives' thought of change as an adventure.

"For example, when Harry S. was told he was being transferred from California to Pennsylvania, he contacted the local tourist bureau in his future town to find out what sights and activities were available. Before the move, he made plans for adventurous weekends there. By the time he and his family made the move, they were anticipating it with enthusiasm."

● *Have a goal in life.* "Goal setting is essential for everyone who wishes to remain healthy under stress," says Dr. Kobasa. "Too many people have only half-formed goals. Highly stressed executives coped with many difficulties when they had set career goals which they considered of such overwhelming importance that they were willing to go through a great deal to accomplish them."

"For example," Dr. Maddi says, "the Smiths were short of cash when they moved into their new home. But they laid out a 'five-year plan,' which included furnishing their house room by room by setting aside a certain amount each week."

● *Have a clear set of personal values.* "This will help you differentiate things which are important from things which are not," advises Dr. Maddi. "If your own set of values places prime importance on a wholesome family relationship, you will not be as frustrated or upset by on-the-job difficulties. You will know that all is well on the home front, where things really matter to you.

"Having your own set of values also includes thinking of yourself as a capable, imaginative, levelheaded individual, as being able to rely on yourself to come through a crisis. This comes about by knowing where you stand on issues of importance—by having a sense of self-identity that does not change easily over time."

● *Have a sense of control over life.* "When things happen to hardy souls, they often feel they can influence the outcome," says Dr. Maddi.

"You can gain this sense of control by developing skills that give you a sense of mastery. When you can fix your own car, sew your own clothes and do minor home repairs, you grow surer of yourself. Maintaining a tight grip on your financial affairs is yet another way of gaining a sense of control in life."

STEP 4: TURN STRESS INTO ENERGY

As you take charge of stress, you can turn it into new energy, which will actually help you achieve your goals, says Dr. Rosalind Forbes, head of a New York consulting firm that teaches top executives how to cope with stress.

Learn to recognize when stress is getting the better of you by watching for the various signals we have already discussed. Then repeat to yourself: "While I may strive for perfection, I'm going to make mistakes. It's only human and I accept this." By doing this, you will realize and accept your own limits.

Assess your goals regularly and set time frames for change. Say: "If this doesn't work, I'll try that after X period of time." Knowing that you have an alternative or a fall-back position can help you cope with difficulties and may serve as a safety valve for frustration. Sometimes, knowing that you don't have to be "stuck" in a situation where you're not seeing any progress can help you hold onto that important sense of being the master of your own destiny.

STEP 5:   LEARN TO RELY ON INSTINCT

"Animals cope with stress more sensibly than humans," says psychologist Dr. Charlotte Tatro. "They can teach us a thing or two." Dr. Tatro, who is director of the Institute for Women at Florida International University in Miami, cites a number of stress-reducing strategies that humans can borrow from the animal world.

● *Seek solace among your loved ones.*   "When danger threatens, many animals instinctively huddle together. Likewise, people under stress should seek the support of those close to them."

● *Give yourself breathing room.*   Many animals don't "invade another herd's territory, nor do they allow theirs to be intruded on." Whenever possible, people should avoid jam-packed, stress-producing situations, such as crowded highways, rush-hour subways and noisy restaurants.

● *Know when to quit.* Animals are not afraid to retreat from a losing battle. But supercompetitive humans tend never to give in and make themselves suffer too much stress as a result.

● *Move away from bad environments.* "Almost every animal species which has survived over many centuries has been wise enough to migrate to a more satisfactory environment when their native habitat no longer provided the food or safety they required." Humans could avoid a great deal of stress by "moving out of uncomfortable situations—an unsatisfactory job, a boring circle of friends, a deteriorating neighborhood."

● *Simplify your life-style when faced with hard times.* When animals face food shortages—"hard times"— they cut down on their birth rate. In a similar way, humans should cut frivolous luxuries in tough economic times to reduce the stressful burden of paying for them.

● *Share the responsibilities of parenthood with your mate.* Many animals do—and it would make for less stress and more harmony among humans, too.

STEP 6: LEARN TO SAY "NO!"

Dr. Robert Eliot, former cardiology consultant to NASA, now chairman of the Department of Preventive and Stress Medicine at the University of Nebraska Medical Center, has long been concerned about the toll stress is taking on our hearts. He wants to cut down on the emotional overreactions people have to everyday problems and suggests that learning to say "no" is a great way to start.

First, imagine that you have just six months to live. Then cut out all the activities you wouldn't bother with. Next, identify stress-causing problems at work and defuse them. Dr. Eliot gives this example: "Let's say your boss piles on the work—more work than you can possibly do—and then gives you an impossible deadline. This is where communication is important. You should go to the boss. Say: 'I enjoy the work I'm doing and I think I do it well, but I can only do so much. I think I've reached my limit.' You know that if you're a good worker, the boss will want to keep you. He will listen to what you have to say."

You can learn to say "no" in other situations as well. Don't agree to do things for friends and others that you don't really want to do—and don't feel guilty about it.

For example, Rose held down a full-time job in addition to the job she had raising her two children alone. Rose's aged father lived a few blocks away, and on the weekends she would clean his apartment, prepare some dishes for the week ahead, do her father's laundry and so on.

But often, when the old man felt the need for some company, he would call Rose at work, or just when she was preparing her family's dinner, and say that he needed some errands to be done. Because she didn't know how to say "not right now" without feeling guilty, Rose pushed herself to the point of exhaustion, trying to take care of everyone in her life.

Finally, when she felt she had no time to rest or enjoy her own life, Rose learned to separate the real emergencies from the chores that could wait—or be done by others. She got her children to pitch in and help entertain their grandfather and to run the odd errands he needed during the week.

STEP 7:   STOP CREATING YOUR OWN STRESS!

"Stress is not an inescapable fact of life, but an emotional reaction to a situation caused by a perception of threat to ego, self-esteem and to our sense of emotional security with people," says Dr. Frank C. Richardson, associate professor of educational psychology at the University of Texas in Austin and coauthor of *Stress, Sanity and Survival*. This is the central theme of a stress management training program Dr. Richardson developed.

Take the following examples of how two people handled a potentially stressful situation in entirely different ways, based on their perceptions:

Jane was hostess at a dinner party for which she had made careful preparations. One of her guests arrived in a sullen, unpleasant mood. As the evening wore on, Jane made a great effort to change her visitor's attitude, to draw him into the conversation and to get him to enjoy himself—but with little result. She ended the evening suffering from a migraine headache and a stomachache, and sick at heart. Inwardly, she felt her guest's displeasure was a negative reflection on her. She felt his unpleasantness proved that she was a basically incompetent, worthless, unattractive human being, who was not skilled or gracious enough to handle a difficult situation.

Susan, faced with an almost identical situation, reacted quite differently. When one of her dinner guests arrived in a foul mood, she was friendly and considerate, but did not try overly hard to entertain him. She assumed he had problems he was not willing to discuss and would probably call the next day to apologize for or explain his behavior.

While the situations both hostesses faced were basically the same, Jane experienced a great deal of stress, while Susan did not. This is Dr. Richardson's point: "We are stressed, not by events, but by the way we view them."

CHANGING YOUR ATTITUDE

"Often there is very little we can do to change disturbing happenings," says Dr. Richardson. "Therefore, the best way to deal with stress and thus avoid many of its dire consequences is to change our view of the world and of the people in it.

"Anger and anxiety, for example, are emotions within our control," he explains. "If you have made arrangements to meet a friend for lunch and she does not show up, you can get angry, believing she is thoughtless, inconsiderate and does not really care for you. Or, you can refuse to get emotionally disturbed, since you have no real basis for reacting that way. You might feel concern for her safety, thinking some accident may have befallen her. The differences in your emotional response are solely the result of the interpretation you choose to place on the situation."

Dr. Richardson emphasizes that most stress-producing ideas can be reduced to a few key mistaken beliefs that we hold about ourselves and the world around us. These mistaken beliefs lead us, he says, "to make cruel and impossible demands upon ourselves and others, and are the root cause of the hurry, frustration and growing sense of hopelessness that often characterize overstressed lives."

An important step toward stress-free living is to give up the superstitious belief that worry will help you prevent mistakes and misfortunes, help anticipate the future or give you added control over the course of events. "Regardless of how many times people have been told that worrying does not accomplish anything, many still believe that active worrying is an essential ingredient in their daily coping abilities. When faced with uncertainty, problems or unfamiliar situations, they can think of nothing more to do than worry.

"People who are anxious most of the time are wedded to the misbelief that worrying keeps them alert to possible danger, or protects them from committing an assortment of errors, and fear that, if they stopped worrying, they would expose themselves to a whole host of possible dangers." Dr. Richardson points out that when things work out badly, people like this often decide it was because they did not worry enough.

To make your life less stressful you must not only give up the worrying habit, he explains, you must also understand why it is useless. There are, he says, only two possible kinds of situations: those we can control or influence in some way and those over which we have no control whatever.

"When you worry about situations you *can* influence, you are draining energy and attention away from the task at hand, which is to develop a problem-solving strategy. When you worry about things over which you have *no control,* you are dwelling on unpredictable and exaggerated, possibly negative, outcomes, which will give you more grief than can possibly be called for."

To overcome the habit of worrying, Dr. Richardson suggests you remind yourself frequently that worry accomplishes nothing. "To avoid needless stress, adopt an attitude which allows you to lose yourself in the process of living. Forget about the past and the future, live mostly in the present and enjoy it."

Stop trying to constantly please others. When you do this, it's based on the mistaken idea that this is the way to get them to like you. The harder you try to do what you believe will make someone else like you, the more stressed you're likely to feel. This is because you rarely get the response you hope for and also end up never doing the things that please you.

To gain people's respect and good wishes without stressing yourself, Dr. Richardson advises that you earn acceptance for yourself, as you are. "To increase your sense of emotional security with people, you must believe that they like you when you are being yourself, not just because you are striving to please them.

"It is not selfish to pursue your own goals, interests and ideas. It is the only way to achieve a sense of purpose in life and to establish yourself in your own and other people's eyes as a worthwhile individual who is dedicated to something outside of himself.

Stop depending on anyone but yourself for happiness. "No other person can make you happy and secure. You must do this for yourself. When you expect others to 'make you happy,' you will suffer frustrations and anxiety, because most people do not think they were put in this world to live up to your expectations or fulfill your needs."

Dr. Richardson explains that it is up to you to "make the most of your opportunities, finding interesting and challenging things to do, so that you are absorbed in meaningful pursuits and activities and no longer have time to waste fretting over your unsatisfactory dependence on anyone else."

When you hold no one but yourself accountable for your own happiness, you will feel far less stress, Dr. Richardson says, "because you will no longer tend to condemn others or find their behavior intolerable, merely because they are not satisfying your needs. You will not feel threatened when they act in their own best interests, and your emotional security will no longer depend on their regard."

Once you gain some insight into your own mistaken beliefs, and once you understand their emotional consequences, you will get a sense of relief that will allow you to live in a more relaxed and tension-free way. And once you start thinking in new ways, you will develop new attitudes that will help you to deal more effectively with stress.

As we have seen in the seven steps toward stress management, you need to change your attitude about stress—you have to alter your behavior and habits. That sounds like a big order, but it isn't. In each step you have seen examples of how to act out the behavior that fits a change in attitude. Let's review the information briefly:

Step 1: Conquer "awfulizing" by controlling the five attitudes of fear, vulnerability, being too demanding, being too judgmental and pessimism. You do this by confronting your fears one small step at a time; ceasing to see yourself as the vulnerable victim and taking control of your life; no longer setting standards that are impossible for you or those close to you to live up to; rethinking your worries to see whether they are real or imagined and too pessimistic; and not finding fault in everyone by judging others too harshly.

Step 2: Change your outlook and count stress as a blessing by realizing that it is alerting you to a problem. Once you understand that stress can help you, you can face the problem and try to solve it.

Step 3: Face the challenge of stress by developing a stress-hardy personality. You can learn to tackle problems, instead of running from them; think of changes in life as adventures; set goals you want to work hard to obtain; establish a clear set of personal values to structure your personal and working life; learn to rely on yourself and your skills to give you the feeling of being in charge of your life.

Step 4: Learn from stress and turn it around by accepting your mistakes and limitations and planning a fall-back strategy if things don't work out as you had planned.

Step 5: Learn from the behavior of animals that you need the support of family and friends; should have enough room to breathe; must give in once in a while; can leave unsatisfactory or uncomfortable situations; should cut back on expenses during financial hard times; and need to share the job of being a parent with your spouse.

Step 6: Say "no" once in a while, when you are faced with more than you can handle or things you just don't want to do socially —and don't feel guilty about it.

Step 7: Stop creating your own stress by worrying constantly, getting upset for no real reason, always trying to please other people and depending on others for your happiness. Stop thinking that worrying will help. Accept yourself as you are, and remember, it's up to you to make the most out of life.

Our next chapter deals with common everyday stresses and how you can change your behavior to cope with them. If you can incorporate into your life the major areas of change just summarized, you will find that much of the stress that saps your energy and emotions can be reduced. If you can make a commitment to try to lighten the load on your shoulders and bring a bit more relaxation and lightheartedness into your day-to-day experiences, there is a good chance you will find you are enjoying yourself more. We need all the strength and energy and stability we can muster to face the big crises of life—death, loss of employment, accidents, disasters. We can't afford to squander our resources on the hundreds of small—and ultimately unimportant—problems that develop daily. Now let's look at a whole menu of situations which life serves up and figure out how best to deal with them.

CHAPTER III

Coping with Family Stress

DO YOU SCREAM AT YOUR KIDS, THROW AN OCCASIONAL plate at the wall, fight with your husband about silly things? Do you wonder why your neighbor doesn't, why she seems always to be on top of things and finds time to cook new recipes when you can hardly cope with hamburgers? Well, there are two possibilities: one is that your neighbor only lets off steam in the privacy of a soundproofed house, the second possibility is that your neighbor has learned how to cope with stress and that she does find more pleasure in her days than you do.

You are probably never going to know for sure what goes on in your neighbor's house. Besides, it would actually be best if you turned your attention back to your own house and tried to get the "true" picture of what's going on there.

Families are little "mini-societies" that serve as hothouses for stress. There are the conflicts between two different generations with different value systems and life-styles living under the same roof; there are power struggles between adult authority and the singlemindedness of teenage "freedom fighters"; there is the struggle inherent in sibling rivalry, where brother and sister fight for attention; and there are the demands of working versus the demands of family life. In essence, it is easy for family members to all feel put-upon, overworked, underloved, neglected. But, it may not be as hard as you think to produce a lot more cheer than anger in your family. There are ways to understand the many moods and currents running through your family, and there are ways to defuse tension that internal and external forces bring to your home. There is behavior which will calm stress and bring it into perspective. The most important thing to remember is that everyone in a family is stressed and that everyone can help take on the responsibility to relieve some of the burden.

SURVIVING THE SUPERWOMAN SYNDROME

It is tough enough when women are expected to be good wives, mothers, homemakers and lovers. There are plenty of women who are not appreciated for the job of running a household and a family. And there are also plenty of women now who have added another job to their already overcrowded schedule; that of money-maker. For whatever reason, a little extra cash or financial necessity, many women are working double shifts—in the home and in the office.

It is not surprising that some women are so over-whelmed with these added responsibilities that they develop a condition known as the "superwoman syndrome." We all know some of the symptoms, including fatigue, stomachaches, headaches, dizziness, high blood pressure, ulcers, anxiety, depression, anger and even thoughts of suicide. It's hardly surprising. Take a look at Dorothy:

Dorothy used to pray every night when she got into bed that she would wake up to a twenty-seven-hour day. She always had a million-and-one things that needed her attention, but which she never got to.

Dorothy would get up at five A.M. every day to get a jump on things. She'd put through two tubs of laundry while she made the kids' lunch, then cook breakfast while she ironed a blouse and skirt for the office and planned the dinner menu. Once the children got up, she sat with them while they ate and looked over their homework. She left her husband Sam his hot meal and went upstairs to dress the children and herself. Sam left for work as she came down the stairs, and, grabbing her bag and coat, Dorothy packed the children in the car and drove them to school.

Once at the office, Dorothy was kept hopping answering phones, typing letters and reports, arranging out-of-town business trips and setting up sales conferences. By the end of the day she was wiped out. She often skipped lunch in order to get off work in time to do the shopping for dinner.

After dinner, Dorothy would take up one of the projects she'd left unfinished from the day before: cleaning, ironing, or clearing out the refrigerator. Pretty soon it was midnight and Dorothy would suddenly realize that Sam had put the children to bed and gone to sleep himself. Often, at this hour of the night, Dorothy would feel sad and depressed without any specific reason. Sometimes she would sit quietly for a few minutes and feel the tears welling up in her eyes. Then she'd shake herself out of it and go to sleep praying for a twenty-seven-hour day.

No wonder Dorothy wanted more time! What she packed into a day would bring most people to their knees in a week. The question is, how do you handle a situation like this? What can be done if you suffer from the exhaustion, tension and ill health of trying to be a superwoman?

Dr. Harold Voth, a psychiatrist and professor of psychotherapy at the famed Karl Menninger School of Psychiatry, offers some expert suggestions on how to beat the problem:

1. Take care of yourself. "Women tend to take care of themselves last, putting their husbands and children first," says Dr. Voth. "Recognize that it's in your family's best interest for you to take care of yourself, both emotionally and physically.

"Many women eat on the run. They don't eat breakfast and they drink gallons of coffee. Do eat breakfast and lunch. Your energy level will be much higher and you won't be running on just nerves. Exercise is a great reliever of stress. Even a brisk half hour walk daily is adequate exercise."

2. Plan your time and effort. "Don't just do things helter-skelter," Dr. Voth advises. "Plan ahead. Don't make three trips downtown when you could make just one."

3. Schedule time for yourself. "Take a scented bubble bath and relax with an inflatable bath pillow behind your head. Read a good book. Have lunch with a friend or coworker," Dr. Voth suggests.

4. Get help. Assign household tasks to your husband and children—or get outside help. Dr. Voth advises: "If you're working out of financial necessity, make it clear that you're working for the sake of the family and you deserve some help."

5. Recognize your limits. You can't strive for perfection in everything. "A woman may not want to lower her standards by asking her husband or children to help with the housework," Dr. Voth says. "But in the long run, she pays a high price for such perfectionism."

THE STRESS-PRONE SPOUSE

Does your spouse always hurry . . . always try to be the best . . . take on too many responsibilities . . . not know how to relax and have a good time?

Does your spouse walk through the door after a long day at work, make dinner, gulp dinner down and then work on household chores until it's time for bed? Is every minute of his or her day heavily scheduled, with not a moment to unwind? Does your spouse think that relaxation is a waste of time—or something to feel guilty about? Is his or her idea of a good time some type of competitive sport or activity?

If your spouse has these characteristics, then he or she is stress-prone—and that high-intensity way of life is probably affecting you and your family. "Stress can be contagious. It can affect everybody in the home," says Dr. Rosalind Forbes, author and stress expert. But you can help relieve the tension generated by a stress-prone spouse and learn to live more happily together by following a few tips from Dr. Forbes:

● Find things you both enjoy and do them together. Attend a wine-tasting class or music appreciation course together. Take a course in ballroom dancing. Rediscover the joys of having fun together. What you do is unimportant—as long as it relaxes both of you.

● Avoid playing any competitive sports with your spouse. Try to get some physical exercise—but do not challenge your stress-prone mate to a tennis or racquetball match. Go bicycling or hiking—just for fun.

● Set aside "free time" for each mate to do whatever he or she pleases. "Find some quiet time each day," says Dr. Forbes, "whether it's a walk after dinner, or just sitting for a few moments. Let your mind wander. Take a mental vacation."

● Trade responsibilities with your spouse. "For example, a husband can offer to take care of the children once a week, so his wife can take a special class or go to a favorite concert." Similarly, a wife can take on one of her husband's usual chores—like taking the family car for servicing or mowing the lawn—so that he can have the luxury of that free time to do whatever he wants.

● Reward your spouse any time he or she stays cool in a tense situation. For example, if your husband tends to blow up when dinner isn't ready on time, or if your wife gets irritable when a kitchen appliance breaks down, take special notice when he or she handles situations like this calmly. The reward can be something simple—like going to a funny movie together or buying a book of jokes and sharing the laughs. The rewards are relaxing in themselves —and they can help your mate stay calm in the future.

● Remind your spouse to live for today, instead of worrying about the past or future. If he or she is constantly preoccupied with mistakes made yesterday or problems that might come up tomorrow, then he or she probably doesn't know how to enjoy life as it's happening. You can set aside some brief time each day to worry about the past or future, to dwell on your worries, leaving you free to spend the rest of your time enjoying the day.

PRESSURE POINTS IN MARRIAGE

Tensions of all kinds are inevitable in marriage. She may dislike his mother, he may get insulted when she reads in bed when he wants to make love. Sometimes these tensions are minor, and sometimes they build, causing real pressure points in a marriage.

Dotty married Angelo, the only son in a big Italian family. He had been doted on by his mother, his grandmother and his sisters. By the time he married at age twenty-six, he had gotten used to having everything done for him.

When Angelo and Dotty started married life, she was appalled by the way he dropped his clothes on the floor, left the bathroom a mess when he showered and got up from the dinner table without picking up a dish or a piece of silverware.

At first, she teased him about being a "prince" and expecting others to wait on him. But two years later, after their first child arrived, she didn't think his attitude was so funny. Often, at the end of the day, she would end up screaming and calling him a "pig," adding, "I'm not your mother!"

Dotty's shouting and nagging got her nowhere. Angelo simply became more stubborn, defending his habits—though sometimes, in quieter moments, he knew that Dotty had a point.

At best, Angelo probably couldn't become a "neat freak," but, by focusing only on this problem and overlooking all the ways in which he was a good husband and a loving father, all Dotty did was generate more stress for herself.

While stresses of this kind can't be completely eliminated, they can be managed, says Dr. Frank A.

Melone, assistant professor of psychology at Penn State University. Try adopting some new changes in your attitude and behavior—both of you!

● Avoid being rigid in your outlook. You can bend to accommodate your spouse's wishes, rather than insisting things always be done your way. In the case of Dotty and Angelo, a little bending on both sides would have reduced his sloppiness to manageable proportions, instead of allowing it to become the subject of regular fights.

● If you fight, fight fairly. When you do argue, as almost all couples do, don't get insulting. Name-calling or hitting your partner verbally with his/her vulnerabilities is a mistake.

● Support your partner's goals and needs. You may feel it's silly to take up Yoga, but, if that's what your spouse wants to do, respect the decision.

● Be committed to your relationship. Realize that entering a marriage is not like buying a car. Don't have the attitude that, if this doesn't work out, you'll try again. If you are fully committed to making your marriage work, you will have the strength and motivation to work problems out.

● Be open and share your desires, dreams and fears with your mate—except when you think your spouse might not be able to handle it. Don't hurt or "punish" your mate by blurting out that you've had sexual fantasies about your family doctor.

● Find out what makes you tick. It makes a happy relationship easier to maintain. When you know your strengths and weaknesses, you'll have more control over your own behavior. And when you have a better understanding of yourself, you can help your partner to understand you.

WHEN BOTH SPOUSES WORK

There's more money when both husband and wife work—but there's also more stress. Scenes like this one can be common:

Sally arrives home, expecting her husband to have cleaned up the breakfast mess, so that she can start dinner. She finds dishes in the sink, clutter around the stove—and her husband not yet home. She feels angry and resentful, as if she's expected to carry the burdens of a two-job family alone. With a knot in her stomach and the start of a headache, she cleans up and starts dinner.

When her husband, Harry, arrives home, he is tired and tense, too. He has had a very bad day, and that is why he is late. Without noticing that Sally is edgy, Harry collapses into a chair and says, "Boy, you wouldn't believe what happened to-day . . ."

Before he can unburden himself, Sally snaps, "You think you're the only one who had a bad day? What about me? I come home wiped out, about to cook *your* dinner—and I find the dishes still sitting here! I can't take this anymore! You're selfish and thoughtless and . . ."

By the time dinner is ready, neither Harry nor Sally has much appetite. Neither one is able to make peace. They go to bed feeling tense and wake up the next morning feeling miserable. Both have let stress get the better of them—and separate them—instead of bringing them closer together.

Here's another example of the kind of stresses that develop when two spouses work:

For the first two years that Jane and Bill were married, she stayed home and kept house. She handled all the household chores, while Bill took care of the family finances, giving Jane a housekeeping allowance every week.

In order to get enough money for a down payment on a house, Jane took a full-time job. Though Bill now helps with the homemaking chores, she still does most of them. Bill still handles the finances, with Jane turning over her paycheck and receiving an allowance each week. She is angry and resentful, because she feels she is stuck with too many responsibilities—and not enough say in financial matters, even though she is contributing her salary.

Both couples have failed to make the kind of adjustments needed in a two-paycheck family. And both are building up the kind of stresses that can seriously damage a marriage.

If you share problems of this kind, you can reduce the friction in your household by following the suggestions of Dr. Sander Latts, associate professor of family studies at the University of Minnesota and Dr. George Rowe, associate professor of human development at the University of Nebraska:

● Share household responsibilities. "If both partners work and one does most of the chores, it builds resentment. The best way to split the household chores is to divide them up on the basis of personal preference," says Dr. Latts. "The ones that neither partner prefers should be split up evenly."

● Discuss money matters openly with your spouse. "With both partners contributing to a paycheck, each should have a say in how the money is being spent," advises Dr. Rowe.

In the case of Jane and Bill, discussions of this kind would easily have resolved the problem. Both were in agreement on the goal of saving for a house. What Jane resented was being treated like a dependent, instead of a partner, a situation that could have been remedied, if she had calmly and rationally voiced her feelings to her husband.

● Plan your time together carefully. All couples can benefit from this advice, but working couples need it especially. Make sure you spend some time every day, perhaps after the children are in bed, talking with each other. This can help nurture your sense of togethership and partnership, in spite of the pressures each of you faces separately during the day.

● Enjoy a night out each week without the children. Again, this is particularly important for working couples, who very often get caught up in their responsibilities and forget how to be sweethearts. And schedule weekends carefully, not haphazardly, so you can spend most of the time with your family. "Husband and wife should arrange to take their vacations at the same time, if possible, because family vacations are a good way to build harmony," Dr. Latts says.

ADJUSTING TO MALE/FEMALE ROLE CHANGES

The changing values of today's world have created many new stresses in marriages. But by making a new series of marital promises, you can lead happier and healthier lives, according to Dr. Carlton A. Hornung, associate professor of preventive medicine and community health at the University of South Carolina School of Medicine.

Sharon and John are a good example of a couple whose marriage has kept pace with changing values.

After John got out of the army, Sharon worked at a job she didn't particularly like to put him through school until he got a degree. When John got settled in his career, Sharon took time off to have a baby. Two years later, she found she missed working—but didn't want to go back to the job she had.

Sharon had always dreamed of becoming a lawyer, but after she married she had given up that goal. John felt that she should have the chance to realize her ambition, especially since she had helped him get started in a career he chose.

Though it wasn't easy, John supported Sharon, financially and emotionally, while she attended law school. He arranged his work schedule so that their young son would not have to spend too many hours a day with a babysitter. Now Sharon has a career she loves—and her marriage to John is stronger and richer than ever.

"If husbands and wives make agreements that promote understanding and equality, they can reduce stress," says Dr. Hornung. "And by reducing stress, we can reduce illness."

Dr. Hornung explains that the changing role of women—including two-career marriages and expanding aspirations of housewives—is introducing new tensions into marriages. These tensions can lead to illness. He reached his conclusions in a massive five-year study of 617 couples which was designed to determine which factors lead to stress, ill health and unhappiness.

Dr. Hornung says that couples must make certain commitments to each other and stick to them. "Learn to live with whatever work the other person is doing. It's very difficult if your spouse is a cab driver or an executive in terms of demand on time, and [in the case of the executive] preoccupation and the need to work at home. Both partners must make adjustments to help cope with threats to the other's job." For example, if your spouse has been promoted to a better, higher-paying job that requires him or her to work longer hours, you will only add to that stress if you begin complaining or acting neglected. On the other hand, if you offer support and assurance, your spouse will be appreciative and your marriage will be less stressed.

"A man should support his wife and her aspirations," says Dr. Hornung. "And he should recognize the frustrations and conflicts women face in trying to realize those aspirations. Men must now help women in their careers, just as women have been helping men."

THE DANGERS OF STRESS AT THE DINNER TABLE

Are scenes like this one familiar at your home?

Mom is preparing dinner, brooding over the note that son Tim has brought home from school—saying that he has failed to bring in three successive homework assignments and that he is in danger of failing.

Dad walks in the door and Mom hands him a stack of unpaid bills as an "appetizer." Before he has a chance to "digest" these, they sit down to eat. Mom begins: "Well, Tim, will you explain to your father why Miss Jones wants to fail you in English?"

Before this family gets through the pot roast and mashed potatoes, each of them has to chew over an unhealthy dose of stress. Stress at meal times is never healthy, but, at the dinner table, it can be particularly dangerous, says cardiologist Dr. William Nelson. "Stress experienced while eating the evening meal is especially damaging to the heart.

"Digesting food places an increased burden upon the heart. When emotional stress is experienced at the same time, there is an increase in blood pressure and heart rate, which may set the stage for eventual damage. When you eat and aggravate yourself, it's like setting off a dangerous charge of TNT in your system. A surprising number of angina pectoris patients have had full-blown heart attacks late in the evening, after they've finished dinner."

Even apparently healthy people are at risk, says Dr. William Nelson, who is professor of medicine at the University of Kansas School of Medicine in Kansas City. He warns: "Millions of people who think they are young and healthy put themselves in danger of becoming future heart attack victims by unsuspected nightly exposure to an emotionally charged dinner hour with their families."

Dr. Nelson offers these suggestions if you want to avoid stress at the dinner table:

● Don't eat as soon as you come home from work. "Every member of the family—mother, father and children—needs a 'quiet time' to make the transition from their daily activities to their relationships with the family," he says. "Schedule dinner at least thirty minutes after everyone has arrived home."

● Start the meal with a simple family ritual, such as saying grace. If you're not religious, you might just join hands for a moment.

● Don't discuss any controversial subjects. In the case of the family we used as an example, it would have been just as convenient—and much healthier—to postpone the unpaid bills and the son's school problems until later in the evening.

"Conversation around the dinner table should be limited to light, noncontroversial topics," says Dr. Nelson. "This is not the time to start bringing up problems."

ARE YOUR CHILDREN INHERITING STRESS?

Parents who are overwhelmed with on-the-job stress are passing emotional problems on to their children, and the kids don't know how to handle it. Do you come home from work and yell at your kids the way your boss yelled at you today? Are you too busy to make time to listen to your child's problems or pick up on his moods of fear or depression? Do you constantly let your children fend for themselves in the afternoons, evenings and weekends?

If you answered yes to any of these questions, you have a lot of company. According to Dr. Perry Buffington, who specializes in treating emotionally disturbed children, and Harvard psychiatrist Dr. William Appleton, there is an "epidemic" of depression among youngsters and much of it is the result of the stress their parents bring home with them. Dr. Buffington says, "What is tragic is that children don't know when their dads and moms are reacting to stress—and they don't know how to handle it."

Dr. Appleton adds: "Many of today's parents are so busy that they expect their kids to go it alone before they're ready. As a result, I am seeing many youngsters experiencing anxiety, confusion and a loss of a sense of self-esteem and confidence." Both experts agree that children should be expected to assume some responsibilities and chores as part of their role in the family, but they shouldn't lose their time to play and be kids.

If you are concerned about your children and want to help them adjust to the stress you and your spouse are under, there are steps you can take. Start with making time for your children. If something interferes with this shared time, explain the problem clearly and make the child feel loved. And, if you feel grumpy after you get home from work, tell your child that you are grumpy because of the hard day's work, not because of him. What if you just explode and yell at your daughter for no reason? Quickly explain that she is not the cause of your anger.

Try to leave your office problems at the office. Try to separate the office from your home life. Be aware of your child's behavior and review how you are handling any discipline problems. And finally, remember that "kids need to be kids," and need time to play, if they are to become well-rounded adults.

YOUR ROLE AS TEACHER

Alice is a housewife and proud of it. She thinks she has a hard job and handles it well—except when the burdens are just too great. Then Alice tells the children to amuse themselves and goes to her bedroom and cries. Sometimes she doesn't come out for hours. But when Alice finally reemerges, she bounces back, cooking dinner and dealing with her children's squabbles with her usual energy. Alice is proud of her personal style of handling too much stress. It works and doesn't hurt the family the way yelling and screaming do.

Or does it? Some experts believe that the way children handle stress is a reflection of the way their parents do. Alice's children may not have to suffer through a temper tantrum, but they are learning that the way to cope is to retreat and ignore the other members of the family. And, while this may be "acceptable" at home in the privacy of the house and family, what is a school principal, camp counselor or boss going to think of such behavior?

Too many parents forget that their children's school teachers are not the only "teachers" in their lives. A child's first and most persuasive teachers are his mom and dad. And kids pick up not only speech, laughter, skills and values, but behavior patterns as well. Think of how enjoyable and gratifying it is when your daughter also likes to cook or sew or dance just as much as you do. Think of the pleasure it gives you when your son likes tinkering with machinery in his spare time, right along side of you. Now think about all your habits you wouldn't want your son or daughter to pick up from you—swearing, driving too fast, drinking, arguing with your neighbor.

Think of two people you know at work or see socially, who seem to have the same skills, backgrounds, education and other characteristics. Do they handle problems in the same way? Or does one explode in rage, while the other uses his energy to solve the problem? Does one attack you personally when he's angry and the other take a break and have a cup of coffee in a quiet corner away from the source of aggravation? There are surely many factors involved in why these two seemingly similar people handle stress differently. But it is a safe bet that a good part of the answer lies in how these individuals were taught by their families to handle stressful events and circumstances.

If you rely on your family and friends to help you handle problems; if you talk out your troubles rather than hiding them; if you have a healthy perspective on what constitutes a big crisis and what is a minor event; and if you have the sense and the strength to deal with the stress in your life effectively—you are providing your child with patterns of behavior he can copy and use to deal with his life. It is a tall order for anyone. No one can be perfect. But we can all try—and what better reason to try than for the sake of our children?

TENSION IN YOUR LOVE LIFE

Which would you rather do, make love or make war? You might be surprised to find that subconsciously you would rather make war, and that's exactly what you do time and time again. By fighting, you can release a lot of the pent-up anger and frustration in your life without having to really open up about what's troubling you. By making love, you can release many of the same tensions and bottled-up energy, but you also have to admit that you need some comforting and closeness. Fighting separates people by pitting them against each other, and one is usually the loser. Loving can bring two people together and substitute communication for combat.

Married or not, you are going to encounter stresses in your love life. These too can be controlled, says Dr. Robert Gordis, author and professor at the Jewish Theological Seminary of America. The first step is to restore communication. "One good way is to watch TV together, then switch off the set and talk about the show you've just seen. Find out each other's opinions, discuss the message in the show or talk about what made you laugh. Do anything that will open communication."

This can be especially helpful if people have been together for a long time and have stopped talking and sharing opinions—or if they're afraid to talk freely about certain topics.

For example, Helen had recognized that Jim was a "quiet," rather withdrawn man from the start of their relationship. She had hoped that once they got to know each other better, he would "open up" and tell her more about himself. However, this didn't happen and Helen began to feel cut off from Jim, in spite of the fact that their relationship was becoming more regular and more "serious" for both of them.

The situation improved greatly when Helen finally realized that Jim was not comfortable about directly revealing his personal thoughts. But she found that she could learn a great deal about him when they talked about movies, stories they had read, people they knew.

It's also important to talk about things that are bothering you, advises Dr. Vincent Foley, psychologist and member of the American Association for Marriage and Family Therapy in New York. "Don't let it build up inside you. Let it out." Verbalizing tensions that are building inside of you prevents you from turning into a pressure cooker, ready to explode, often at inappropriate times. This doesn't mean you should snap at your partner every time you feel a minor irritation, but rather that you should find ways to make your needs known in a nonthreatening way.

For example, Claire felt that the success of her relationship with Stan, a somewhat domineering, opinionated man, lay in deferring to him, no matter what she thought. But every so often, the pressure of all the things she never said would build up in Claire, and she would explode into a temper tantrum over some relatively minor remark. Stan would be totally bewildered by these outbursts, which seemed to come out of "left field," and, lacking any other explanation, he put them down to "female nerves."

These temper tantrums weren't helpful to either Stan or Claire. She would end up feeling foolish and weak. It would have been far better if Claire allowed herself to express her thoughts when she disagreed with Stan.

Another valuable stress-reducer is to recognize the importance of freedom in a relationship. People in love wrongly believe that they should do everything together, says Dr. Foley. "They end up suffocating each other, and this becomes a prime breeding ground for stress. Freedom is extremely important in reducing stress. Spend time away from each other. Developing interests independent of each other will breathe fresh life into any relationship suffering from stress."

Sometimes people who have been together for a long time will hesitate to pursue independent interests, because they are afraid their partners will feel hurt, neglected or threatened. But if these outside interests can be approached in a nonthreatening way, by assuring one another that the relationship is still very important, then both partners can feel secure enough to enjoy occasional "breathers" from one another.

Rosemary had been brought up by her mother to believe that a neglected husband will "stray," so that even after nine years of marriage, she still planned to spend most of her leisure time with Jerry.

But one day, while they were discussing some of their problems in a frank and open fashion, Jerry confessed that he had mistaken her attentiveness for dependency and that he had found her "Siamese-twins" notion of marriage oppressive.

After the two of them felt confident and secure enough to spend time away from each other, to develop personal friends and interests, they found that they bickered less and enjoyed one another more.

Another way to control stress is to avoid accusing your partner of things that he or she has no control over, says Dr. Gordis.

In stress-filled marriages, you will hear things like: "YOUR mother is impossible," or "YOUR son is driving me crazy." Statements like this only inflame stress.

And finally, remember to respect the needs and rights of your partner.

RELEASING ANGER CAN BE BAD FOR YOU

Popular wisdom tells us that releasing anger is healthy, that suppressing it can be dangerous to health. But experts now say there is no evidence to support this idea; that, in fact, just the opposite is true.

People who explode with anger as a means of "getting it off their chests" are actually risking more stress and hypertension than those who swallow their anger, says psychiatrist Dr. William Appleton.

"Your body can suffer more from expressing anger to, say, your wife than it would if you tried to overlook the problem, changed the subject and didn't dwell on it," says Dr. Appleton, assistant clinical professor of psychiatry at Harvard Medical School. "After expressing extreme anger, most people are very, very sorry. They don't feel better; they feel remorseful, guilty and upset. That's a form of stress, and stress can lead to things like hypertension."

Dr. Richard Proctor, professor and chairman of the department of psychiatry at Bowman Gray School of Medicine, Wake Forest University, agrees. "Sometimes, if you ventilate hostility, you're going to feel guilty about it, and that may cause more problems. Plus, you may get more hostility back—and then you have a Ping-Pong game."

HOW SEX CAN REDUCE TENSION

Picture this scene:

Nina has just had "words" with a neighbor who allows his dog to leave all kinds of messes in her backyard. The neighbor is not cooperative and counters Nina's complaint with a threat to call the police next time Nina and her husband play their stereo past ten o'clock.

Nina's husband, Robert, has had his share of problems, too. He has just heard a rumor that his company is going to be cutting costs by phasing some departments out. He is afraid that his department will be the first to go.

When he gets home, Nina can see he's troubled, so she doesn't bother him with the neighbor problem. They have dinner, and later they discuss Robert's worries and Nina's encounter. Talking about their troubles makes them both feel better.

But both feel the need of some extra "tender loving care." They put some romantic music on the stereo, open a bottle of wine—and spend the next hour making love.

Robert and Nina have discovered an important secret for staying healthy. "Unhurried, passionate sex is better for your health than 100 sit-ups, tiger's milk or a visit to a health spa," says Dr. Judith Meyerowitz, a New York psychologist associated with Yeshiva University.

Dr. Humphry Osmond, clinical professor of psychiatry at the University of Alabama, agrees, adding "Nothing can replace a close, intimate and passionate relationship. It's worth more than money, more than fame and more than occupational success. It is certainly good for your health." There is a difference, he says, between passionate love and a casual sexual relationship. "You might get physical relief from a stranger, but the intensity is not there—and therefore the physical benefits aren't as intense."

The kind of nurturing, healing effects that Nina and Robert experience when they make love are not found in a casual encounter with a stranger who doesn't really care about you.

Dr. Elaine Hatfield, head of the University of Hawaii

psychology department, notes that: "The better the relationship, the better the health of a couple. Passionate love is good because your hormone levels change and you secrete adrenaline. There is much evidence that this higher level of arousal is good for memory and also keeping your body toned." Best of all, the pleasures and benefits of good sex do not have to diminish with age. Says Dr. Hatfield: "Experts think that after twenty years of marriage, passion increases."

Hidden Sources of Stress

Even if you are especially sensitive to the stresses in your life and your family's, there are times and conditions you've probably never thought of as tension producing. Can your house ever be too clean? Can the end of Christmas madness mean the "blues"? Does a change in the weather mean trouble for your family?

A HOUSE THAT'S TOO CLEAN CAN BE BAD FOR YOUR FAMILY

If you're a fanatic about dust and disorder, your intolerance for messiness can create tension and arguments between you and your family—and make your mate and children uncomfortable in their own home, says a Rutgers University psychologist. Arnold A. Lazarus advises that "the secret is moderation. A little bit of disarray is good for you." Apparently, people can stand different amounts of messiness and the problems come up when couples have widely differing tolerance levels. If you can't stand a smudge on the windowpane or dust on the light bulbs, you had better ask yourself these questions, says Lazarus:

Is a spotless house worth making my family and friends uncomfortable?

Is it worth the constant fights and arguments that arise when I blow up over a dirty sock lying in the living room?

Do I really want my loved ones to be constantly on edge, worrying about getting the house a little messy?

If you answer honestly, you'll probably admit that your family is more important than your house. It takes a little reprogramming, but, if you can let the dinner dishes sit on the table and then reward yourself for doing it by treating yourself to a movie, eating some chocolates or going window-shopping at the local mall, you can begin to change your attitude. Lazarus says that "by rewarding yourself you are psychologically telling yourself that it's all right to live with some untidiness. It's simply a question of reducing friction, tension and arguments by raising your tolerance for untidiness. You are making yourself easier to live with. And you are making your house a home that people can enjoy living in."

SURVIVING POST-HOLIDAY BLUES

Can you believe it? No more standing in line to get Tommy a tractor-trailer set. No more hand-to-hand combat over the last Cabbage Patch doll. You have wrapped the last package, made the last turkey dinner for twenty and silenced the last family argument over whose game it really is. Peace and quiet. Happiness is looking across the room and not seeing a Christmas decoration anywhere. Or is it?

The letdown after the final gift is opened and the

Christmas tree is dismantled can mean trouble for everyone. For married couples it can be a particularly difficult and stressful time, says marriage counselor Dr. Ray Fowler.

"There is an awful lot of postholiday recrimination and bickering," says Dr. Fowler, executive director of the American Association for Marriage and Family Therapy. "Most marriages get into trouble after the holidays. People come down off the high of the holiday season and things start getting off track."

There are several reasons for this postholiday stress. A major one of these is the tendency that many couples have to overspend during the holidays, adds Dr. James Kilgore, president of the Northside Counseling Center in Atlanta. "When the bills start rolling in after the holidays, couples realize they've overstepped their bounds. This puts strain on their marriage. One partner often blames the other for overspending."

Another problem in many marriages is that couples feel depressed because the Christmas spirit has dwindled. "The big family dinners, visiting relatives and friends, the joy of giving and receiving gifts have all slipped into the past," says Dr. Kilgore. "They let the feeling of togetherness and Christmas spirit die too quickly, so they get depressed and end up taking it out on each other."

Further stress comes from the sudden drop in activity after the holidays, Dr. Fowler explains. "During the holidays, people were so busy, they didn't have time to get on each other's nerves."

Dr. Fowler suggests that these feelings are compounded because postholiday weeks are often accompanied by miserable weather, which inhibits many activities.

The experts offer the following tips to help your marriage survive this period of postholiday blues:

● Don't blame each other for overspending. Realize you both went overboard a little and will work together to find ways to pay all the bills.

● Set up a six-month budget to pay back the money you owe. Set a common goal and work it out together.

● Return any gifts you don't need. Don't be embarrassed. By returning the unnecessary items, you can get the things you really need or use the money to pay off your own debts.

● Extend the holiday spirit of togetherness. Get the relatives together one weekend a month for a big turkey dinner or a family activity.

● Make a special effort to visit your friends. You saw old friends during the holiday season, so why wait until next year? Maintain close ties with them.

● Get back into a routine that includes plenty of activity. Don't wait for boredom to set in. Jump right back into your regular activities that you had postponed because of the holiday rush. Go bowling, attend sewing class or whatever other activity you might have been doing before the holidays.

EVEN WEATHER CAN AFFECT YOUR MOOD

Remember last summer when you sweltered day after day? The fans never really cooled you off, and the air conditioning either didn't work on the hottest days or was too costly to run. Remember when you promised yourself that, if it ever got cold again, no matter how freezing you were, you'd never complain? "Give me some relief from the heat," you said, "and I'll never whine again about how blue my toes are turning or how my nose feels like an iceberg when I am lying in bed at night!" Hah! Three weeks into the winter and already you're dreaming of iced tea and sandy beaches, soft summer breezes and shorts and bathing suits!

Changes in your environment—changes in weather—produce stress. And winter can be a particularly stressful time for many people. But you can beat the pressures brought on by cold weather with these tips from a team of experts that included: Dr. Irwin Ziment, professor of medicine at UCLA; Dr. Fred Rohles, director of the Institute for Environmental Research at Kansas State University; Dr. Nelson Hendler, assistant professor of psychiatry at Johns Hopkins University in Baltimore; Dr. Donald Dudley, clinical professor of neurological surgery at the University of Washington; and Dr. Raj Muragali, staff psychiatrist at the Manhattan Psychiatric Center in New York City.

1. "Summerize" your home. Use bright, vibrant colors and cheerful flowered patterns throughout your house. Hang plants and arrange vases of colorful flowers, either real or artificial, wherever you can. Put pictures of warm, tropical places, like Hawaii, on the walls. Also, brighten up a dark, gloomy winter day by turning on more lights. Use light bulbs with a higher wattage than you usually do.

2. Eat summer foods. Prepare a picnic meal of hot dogs, potato chips and ice cream. Or try the kind of spicy foods eaten by people in warm places like Mexico or Spain.

3. Perk up your wardrobe. When you're indoors, wear bright, cheerful clothes, such as floral shirts and white slacks.

4. Cut down the stress of driving. Plan your trips more carefully, taking the weather and the wet, icy roads into consideration. Allow yourself plenty of extra time to get where you're going. Schedule alternate dates for meetings in case of bad weather. Be sure to winterize your car by stocking the trunk with anti-freeze, a good spare tire and even chains. Also, keep things like a thermal jacket, extra gloves, a spare umbrella, raincoat and a flashlight with good batteries in the car.

5. *Prepare your home for bad weather.* Keep candles, electric fuses and a flashlight on hand in case of a power outage.

6. *Relax with warm baths.* Stretching out in a nice hot bath with bubbles or bath oil will soothe your nerves and lift your spirits.

7. *Watch cheerful movies on TV.* Choose light, cheerful films, such as comedies and musicals. Look for movies with summery or tropical settings. Films like these will cut down the stress from feeling depressed about the winter weather outside.

8. *Take care of your health.* Eat plenty of fruits and vegetables during the winter months. Take vitamin and mineral supplements, particularly vitamin C. If you haven't been out in the sunshine, take vitamin D supplements in moderate doses of about four hundred units a day.

9. *Pay special attention to your skin.* Cold, blustery weather can be harmful to your complexion. Also, wind can dry the skin and bring on chill sores. Blemished skin can cause emotional stress, particularly to women, although men can benefit from pampering their skin during winter, too. Apply moisturizer fortified with vitamins, such as A, D and E. When the weather is bad, cover your face as much as possible.

10. *Avoid crowded shopping malls.* Avoid the stress from crowds—particularly during holiday shopping periods—by scheduling your shopping trips for non-peak periods.

11. *Stock your cupboards.* Keep a good supply of canned and frozen foods during the winter months. In

this way you won't be caught without anything to eat on a stormy day—and you can avoid the stress of having to make an emergency trip out during a storm.

12. Organize group activities. When you're cooped up for a long period of time due to bad weather, play some games—such as charades or Monopoly or Scrabble. These can help you cut down on the stress of "cabin fever," which develops when people are shut up together for long periods of time.

13. Plan for the future. Making plans can bring your anxiety levels down, so keep yourself busy with social activities and projects for the future. This is much better than staying home during the cold, dark winter months and brooding about your problems.

14. Schedule vacations for winter. If possible, schedule a vacation in a warmer climate during the winter period—and avoid at least some cold weather.

15. Take one-minute "trips." On cold, dreary days, take brief mental "vacations" by imagining yourself in warm, sunny places.

16. Head off financial problems. It's easy to start feeling financial stress. The holidays can drain your savings, and it can be expensive to heat your home, winterize your car and home and keep your family in winter clothes. To avoid this stress, try to put away a little money for the postholiday season. Another good idea is to use the long winter nights to think of ways to supplement the family income. For example, you and your family can plan summer garage sales or other pleasant money-making activities.

HOW YOU EAT AND DRESS CAN CREATE STRESS

We've all probably heard the slogan "dress for success!" And the rhyme "an apple a day keeps the doctor away!" has been drilled into our heads since childhood. Now, a team of Boston University experts tells us that the clothes we wear and the way we eat can cause stress.

The team consists of Dr. Sanford I. Cohen, chairman of the division of psychiatry at the Boston University's School of Medicine; Dr. Lyle H. Miller, Ph.D., professor of psychiatry and chairman of the department of biobehavioral sciences at the School of Medicine; and Dr. Robert N. Ross, Ph.D. a science and medical author and former director of the University's graduate program in science communications. They have found that, if your clothes fit too tightly, you're subject to both physical and emotional stress. And if you don't establish a regular eating schedule, physical stress is the result.

Tight-fitting clothes prevent the body from assuming its natural posture. Women's high heels are real troublemakers. They throw the body off balance and put heavy stress on the muscles of the legs and back. They also stress the bones, muscles and ligaments of the feet.

Tight clothes worn by both men and women prevent easy bending, moving or turning. Worse, they interfere with normal breathing through the diaphragm and force us into chest breathing.

As babies, we breathed naturally, with the belly going up and down with each breath. But the social pressure of wearing stylish clothes has forced us to keep our bellies still while moving our chest to draw breath.

This is a dangerous habit, because it causes severe physical and emotional stress. For example, some scientists argue that the frightening condition called agoraphobia—panic at the thought of leaving secure, enclosed spaces—is rooted in breathing problems. And cases of agoraphobia have been cured by teaching the patient how to breathe properly.

Agoraphobia is more common among women than men, and that's because women are chest-breathers, due to their tight-fitting clothes. They take shallow breaths; and when they are pushed into situations they find upsetting, they breathe even faster, because their bodies need more oxygen. The result—a panic attack.

Eating habits can be another potent source of stress. If we don't establish regular mealtimes, the body does not know when it is going to get the food that it requires. Physical stress is the result.

If we neglect to keep a regular time schedule for meals, the levels of blood sugar and other necessary substances fluctuate so wildly that the body does not work efficiently. And, in addition, it is also important to chew food thoroughly, since this forces a person to slow down and relax.

AVOIDING STRESSFUL HOME ENVIRONMENTS

Maybe you have a favorite easy chair that, when you flop down into it, makes you feel like a kid again—safe in the lap of your mother or father. Or perhaps it's your bed that's like an island refuge in a tumultuous sea of conflict and aggravation. Wherever you find solace or comfort, it isn't foolish or something to be ashamed of. In fact, it makes perfect sense, according to two sociologists. Your home and its furnishings refresh you after the stresses of a long day—or they can be sources of unnecessary stress in your family.

Atlanta sociologist Dr. Jackie Boles maintains that the type of home a family lives in and the way it's decorated is directly related to the amount of stress in the family. "I've found that marital difficulties and family dissension stem from a stressful home environment," says Dr. Boles, associate professor of sociology at Georgia State University.

"Many people fail to realize the many ways in which their home and its furnishings cause them undesirable pressure. A home can seem completely adequate for a family, but still have an adverse effect on their daily lives."

Dr. Charlotte Tatro, a sociologist at Florida International University in Miami, agrees. "There are many frequently overlooked sources of stress in a family's home environment which can cause jangled nerves, irritability and bad tempers," she says.

"When they remain uncorrected over time, the family develops a hypersensitivity to run-of-the-mill problems, which tends to lead to flare-ups and harsh words. But most of these stress-producing conditions can be overcome easily and inexpensively, once identified."

The two sociologists highlight the following situations as those most likely to cause unnecessary stress on family members:

1. *Living in a home that's too large or too small.*
Young families, for example, may buy a large home, plan to grow into it and then find that the expense and effort required to furnish and maintain the house creates stress.

After two years of marriage, Linda and Phil put a down payment—every penny they could scrape together—on a rambling five-bedroom Victorian house. They reasoned that this would be a great place to raise the children they planned to have—and that the house would turn out to be a great investment after they fixed it up.

However, after they moved the furnishings from their one-bedroom apartment into the house, Linda and Phil found it felt more like a warehouse than a home, with many of the rooms standing empty and bare.

The "fix-up" also turned out to be much more than they could handle, since both of them worked and had little time for "do-it-yourself" projects. They began to quarrel regularly about whose fault it was that they got stuck with such a "white elephant."

Fortunately, they did realize that they had made a mistake and were able to resell the house and move into a much more manageable and "cozy" place.

A longtime married couple whose children have grown up and left home may also have problems with a too-large home, as they rattle around in too much space, feeling lonely, neglected and left behind. For them, the solution could be the adventure of "starting over" together, choosing a new place that feels just right for their new needs.

In a home that's too small, lack of privacy is often the stress-producing element, regardless of the ages of the family members living there. No matter how well family members get along, they do need a place where they can entertain friends, pursue their hobbies—or just be alone—without intruding on anyone else, or being intruded upon.

● If your home is too large, close off unused rooms. Use them for storage, or just pretend they don't exist.

● If your home is too small, clear out the nonessentials to improve the traffic flow. And when you replace furniture, buy smaller pieces. Don't fill every corner with a lamp, chair or table.

2. *Living in a "different" house.* The family who selects a house that is too different—too big, too small, too old, too new, too modern or too traditional—from the rest of the houses in the neighborhood will find that being a misfit creates stress.

• So, if you're buying a new home, don't buy one that seems to be out of step with the rest of the neighborhood.

3. *Picking the wrong room colors*. A small room painted a dark color will seem smaller and more confined, which can create stress. On the other hand, a large room painted a pale color seems larger, and those in it will feel alone and isolated—which can cause stress.

• Small rooms should be papered or painted in light pastel colors, so they'll feel intimate, rather than threatening. And large rooms should be papered or painted in the warmer colors, such as yellow, orange and red.

4. *Exposure to too much noise*. Doors that squeak and slam, appliances that whir and buzz, bare floors that echo every sound—these and other things that create noise can cause family stress.

• Oil squeaking doors and put doorstops on those that slam; put noisy appliances on rubber pads and keep them in good repair so they'll operate more quietly; cover bare floors with throw rugs or a carpet, and do anything else you can to keep noise to a minimum.

TELLING LIES CAN MAKE YOU SICK

After six years of marriage, Joanne had started an extramarital affair with a man who worked in her office. Using a variety of excuses, from "working late" to "dinner with the girls," she was able to keep her husband from finding out.

But each time she was out with her lover, and just before she went home, Joanne would begin to feel anxiety, sometimes bordering on panic. As she mentally rehearsed the lies she would tell her husband, the anxiety would mount, her palms would begin to sweat and her heart would thump faster and faster in her chest.

In time, the lying, compounded by the stresses of the affair, made Joanne a nervous wreck. For the first time in her life, she began to use tranquilizers and to take more than her usual single "social" drink.

Joanne's symptoms are not surprising, for, as experts tell us, lying can be stressful and harmful to your health.

"Lying has been found to be extremely stressful," says Dr. Jaime Quintanilla, clinical professor of psychiatry at the Texas Tech University Health Sciences Center in Amarillo. "The average, normal man or woman cannot tell even a small 'white lie' without shocking every nerve cell in the body."

Lying, he says, triggers the release of hormones that raise the heart rate, blood pressure and respiration. "It also decreases the production of white blood cells, which temporarily weakens one's defenses against all forms of disease."

"The accumulated stresses of lying," Dr. Quintanilla explains, "combined with everyday anxieties and tensions, can so weaken the individual that he may suffer from any number of ailments—such as high blood pressure, ulcers, infections, headaches, insomnia . . . If you tell enough lies, it can make you sick."

Dr. Harold Voth, senior psychiatrist at the Menninger Foundation in Topeka, Kansas, observes: "The very fact that lie detectors work is evidence there is a definite physical stress reaction that accompanies lying. That's what lie detectors measure: stress, the racing heart, sweaty palms, quickened breathing.

"Each time you tell a lie, you give yourself a blow to the body. Repeated too often, this can be both mentally and physically crippling for you. Honesty is not only the best policy for moral reasons, it is also the healthiest way to live."

BOREDOM IS THE HANDMAIDEN OF STRESS

Contrary to popular opinion, it is not necessarily the hard-driving executive who suffers from on-the-job stress. It may well be the assembly-line worker who performs the same task all day long.

Experts say that underwork is one of the chief causes of on-the-job stress—because it leads to dissatisfaction and resulting tension.

"Boring jobs seem to be the hardest on health," revealed Dr. John R.P. French, who conducted a university study on stress. He noted that "high blood pressure, sleeplessness, fast heartbeat, loss of appetite, anxiety, tension and depression" are associated with "jobs where there is too little action, not enough responsibility or decision-making and confusion about roles and titles."

Conversely, he noted that "the eager beaver who puts in long hours, carries a heavy work load and bears a lot of responsibility reports the greatest satisfaction with his job."

And the assembly-line worker isn't the only one who suffers from drudgery. A hamper full of laundry, a floor that needs mopping, a houseful of beds that need making—all these can make you feel harried and pressured and bored. Yet, when it's done right, housework can actually help you relieve stress.

"There are things women can do around the house that help thwart the physical and emotional problems that accompany stress," says Janice Sorlien, associate director of the Stress Resource Institute. The key is to come up with different ways to break up the monotony which often causes stress.

Here are some of Sorlien's suggestions for making household chores a lot more than just drudgery:

Once or twice a week, try a brand new recipe— something you've never cooked before. Instead of preparing the same meals over and over again, make cooking an adventure.

To make laundry seem less tedious, start folding clothes differently. Switch your laundry hours around so that you can do the wash while watching TV at night. Make a deal with your husband so that, once a month, he does the laundry and you wash the car.

When washing the windows, let your imagination wander. Use the window as a looking glass into fantasy land. Fantasy is more than a temporary escape from reality—it's also a good way to release stress.

Even grocery shopping can be made more enjoyable —and less stressful—by approaching it as an outing. First, treat yourself to a meal away from the house. Then take a completely different route to the store.

From time to time, change your entire daily work schedule by turning it upside down. If you usually make the beds first, do them last instead. And in the middle of your housework, do something different and fun— have coffee with a neighbor, spend thirty minutes reading a new book or even take a bubble bath in the middle of the day.

Finally, while you're in the middle of beating a rug or washing the blinds, keep in mind that you could be reaping some physical and emotional benefits far beyond a clean house.

GARDENING AS THERAPY

Do you wrestle with your philodendron, tangle with your ivy or wallop your jade tree? Do you think talking to your plants means talking fast and mean? Is the "easy listening" music in your house easier to listen to from outside because the roar of rock is deafening enough to literally knock the begonias off their saucers? Well, hold on a minute! Stop treating your little potted friends like the undergrowth of the Amazon jungle. That Swedish ivy you love to hate could be helping you—if you'd only give it a chance.

Puttering in a garden, planting seeds and watching them grow, raising vegetables or arranging flowers can be a pleasant and easy way to reduce stress, anxiety and tension. Many universities now offer courses in "horticultural therapy," and professionals in this field are moving into jobs in nursing homes, mental hospitals and prisons.

"Working with plants offers many positive payoffs—it simply melts away stress and anxiety," says Dr. P Diane Relf, assistant professor of horticulture at Virginia Polytechnic Institute and State University. "It' an incredibly wonderful outlet for creativity, and unlike art or music, you can eat what you create Preparing the soil, planting a seed and watching it grow offers everyone a great sense of pride and accomplishment.

"Anytime you feel anxious or angry, I suggest you start puttering with your plants. You'll get instan relief, as your thoughts and deeds are redirected to your plants and away from the source of your stress

Try it, you'll like it. It's better than stuffing yourself with sweets."

The first rule in horticulture is to start small, advises Dr. Relf. You can always expand your garden later. Then decide what kinds of plants you want to grow: flowers, vegetables or houseplants. You can even buy books on the subject, visit garden shows and join a local garden club or plant society.

Coping with the World At Large

We have talked a lot about the stresses inside marriage and the family; how to handle two careers in the same household; kids and how they learn to cope; love as a source of solace. And we've seen some of the unusual sources of stress which, like boredom, lying and the letdown after Christmas, can disrupt the harmony of your life. Now let's turn to some of the stresses of day-to-day living which can make you crazy, unless you learn how to adapt your behavior to cope with the fickleness of life, as well as the demands of the outside world.

WORRYING ABOUT TIME CAN RUIN YOUR HEALTH

"Hurry up, George! It's five past six and we're due at the Wilsons' in two minutes. What on earth is taking you so long?" Harriet is having an attack of the crazies. George is ALWAYS late. They never get anywhere on time, and Harriet is the kind of person who simply CANNOT STAND being late.

George, on the other hand, can never understand

what all the rush is about. In business, he always tries to be on time for appointments, get his reports done on schedule and never keeps his boss waiting. But in his social and personal life George just can't see how it will matter if they get there a few minutes late. "After all," George says, "doesn't every hostess dread that first ring of the door bell—that moment when poor Mrs. Wilson, for instance, will say 'Oh no, they're early!'"

Harriet, however, is downstairs fuming and nearly in tears. "In twenty years of marriage we've never once been on time to a party!" she says to herself. "If George really cared about me, he wouldn't do this to me every single solitary time we go anywhere." Harriet is full of resentment. In her daily activities she is always punctual. If she has agreed to have a cup of coffee with a neighbor, for example, and finds that she is running late with her cleaning, Harriet always drops what she's doing and rushes to get next door right on time. Or when she's meeting some friends for lunch, Harriet will leave twenty minutes earlier than she has to, just so a sudden traffic jam doesn't make her late. In fact, Harriet schedules everything right down to the minute. Everything except George, that is.

"Now it's no longer a question of 'going to be,' George," she yells up the stairs. "Now, we are late. We are late again, and I would rather not go at all than show up late."

Harriet has become a slave to the clock. You've met her a dozen times: she's always glancing at her watch even in the middle of lunch. She looks preoccupied all the time, and, when she relates a story, she has the times down pat, such as: "At 6:15, no make that 6:18, the bell of the stove timer went off, and I knew if we waited another seven or eight minutes the dinner would be ruined." It may be annoying to others, it may seem funny, but it sure isn't healthy to run your life centered around the clock.

If you are the sort of person who checks your watch every few minutes, or, if you drive yourself to be superpunctual, you may be a candidate for serious stress, says Dr. Joseph Nowinski, Ph.D., director of health services at the University of Connecticut.

"Medical experts now believe that chronic watch- and clock-gazing can be a major cause of stress-related illness—and even heart disease," he explains. "And one of the most important stress factors is trying to be punctual to the minute."

Dr. Meyer Friedman, director of the recurrent coronary prevention project at San Francisco's Mt. Zion Hospital, agrees that clock-watching can cause stress when you're "struggling to accomplish too many things in too little time."

To ease the pressures of time, Dr. Nowinski suggests not wearing your watch, leaving it home for a few days. You may be surprised to find how well you can survive without it. You can always ask those around you the time. If you must wear your watch, operate on a time lag. Set the watch fifteen minutes ahead. You'll have a little leeway when you need it.

Stretch your time schedule, Dr. Nowinski advises. People experience stress when they cut corners and don't allow enough time to do things. If you know that getting up at 7:39 A.M. gets you to work at 8:30, try getting up at 7. By having more time to shower, dress and have a bite, you won't start off the day in a stressful rush.

Make your appointments flexible. Instead of saying you'll arrive at a specific time, say you'll be there "around four o'clock" or "fourish." That gives you at least fifteen minutes in either direction.

Schedule timeless days, says Dr. Nowinski. If your work schedule is too rigid to be changed, leave weekends free and flexible. Plan to do things on the spur of the moment.

Don't push the panic button when you're running late. If you're going to be late, face it. But don't start rushing around to the point where you'll make your situation worse by spilling coffee on your clothes.

Slow down. Try to relax. One good trick is to imagine the people waiting on the other end. They know that things like traffic jams can slow people down, and they will understand.

Dr. Alan I. Levenson, chairman of the psychiatry department at the University of Arizona College of Medicine, offers some additional tips:

Set your priorities. Organize your days around the most important things. "Housewives shouldn't try to do all their household chores at once." And don't make yourself feel more rushed by making unrealistic commitments. "Don't tell your boss that you'll have a job done by Wednesday—when you know that's an absolute impossibility."

Stay healthy. "Get enough sleep and eat right. The healthier you are, the less tired you'll feel—and if you're less tired, you'll feel less rushed."

Also, don't try to do two things at once. "Unless you're an absolute whiz at math, don't watch TV and attempt to do your taxes at the same time." And try to make your surroundings at work as comfortable as you can. "When you're comfortable, you work best and feel less rushed."

Harvard psychiatrist Dr. William Appleton is convinced that people who worry about time constantly—who fret about wasting it, losing it or who brood that "time is running out"—are suffering from a life-threatening ailment called "hurry sickness."

"It's a major underlying cause of the entire range of chronic and degenerative diseases, including heart disease, ulcers, high blood pressure and possibly even cancer," says the medical school professor. "People with 'hurry sickness,' as a group, get sick more easily and die earlier. They're susceptible to every type of stress-related ailment, because all illness is affected in some way by a person's sense of time."

"People with 'hurry sickness' are easy to spot," Dr. Appleton adds. "They can't sit still. They fidget, bounce, fret when confined to a chair. Their hands, fingers and feet keep moving. There's a sense of urgency about them. They run late all day long."

"Hurry sickness" is an actual illness, Dr. Appleton insists. "People who are 'time sick' have increased heart rate and high blood pressure, plus elevated levels of hormones normally excreted in large amounts in response to stress.

"They also have increased gastric acid secretions, blood cholesterol, respiratory rate and muscle tension. These are conditions which make people prone to coronary artery disease—the most frequent cause of death."

Dr. Appleton cites a study at a major hospital which showed that heart attack patients who expressed the fear of "not enough time left" had a lower rate of survival. Cancer patients who react with panic to the thought of time running out die earlier than others too, he notes.

Dr. Appleton gives some additional advice for people who suspect they're suffering from the "hurry sickness."

● *Reset your mental clock.* "As you go about your daily tasks, clock yourself. Know how long it takes to finish specific chores."

● *Lighten your load.* Find ways to relieve time pressure. Learn how to say, "No, I don't have the time" when people disrupt your work.

If, for example, you find that stopping to help your fellow workers always leaves you running behind, say, "I'd like to stop and help you, but I really must finish what I'm doing."

Or, if your household chores are constantly being interrupted by a too-friendly neighbor, who wants to chat on the phone or come by for a cup of coffee, say, "I'd love to visit with you, but it will have to wait until I'm finished with my chores."

And stop trying to do everything yourself. It's no admission of failure to say "I need help with this or that."

● *Stop running from unhappiness.* Some people are in a constant rush, because they are afraid to "light" and face a problem that is making them unhappy.

Jennie was a good example of this. She had become very unhappy with her marriage of eighteen years. She felt that the problems were insoluble, that a divorce was the only answer—yet she was desperately afraid to try life on her own. So, instead of facing the source of her unhappiness, she threw herself into her work and into her hobbies with a vengeance, creating such a breakneck pace that she would be literally "too busy to think."

Not only did this fail to resolve her problems, it also made her more tense, more nervous. She began to suffer from headaches and insomnia, until her family doctor insisted she seek counseling to work out her problems and protect her health.

"If your unhappiness is due to an irreplaceable loss—the death of a loved one or the irreversible loss of health—work out your unhappiness with tears and by talking out your feelings with someone else," Dr. Appleton advises.

● *Master your ambition.* "Become involved in stimulating and noncompetitive activities simply for the joy of doing them," he says. "One day, every two weeks, walk more slowly, talk more slowly, eat more slowly, take a longer bath. Get to know your family better. Take long walks or have heart-to-heart talks with all those you love."

HOW TO RELIEVE THE TEDIUM OF WAITING

You don't have to suffer from "hurry sickness" for waiting to get on your nerves. Waiting in traffic jams, crowded stores, doctors' offices and other places is a fact of life. But, when that waiting becomes stressful, it also becomes a health hazard, according to Dr. Thomas L. Saaty, a professor at the University of Pittsburgh Graduate School of Business and a specialist on the effects of waiting.

"People who are waiting become pressured. They feel frustration, anger, helplessness," says Dr. Saaty, who estimates that the average person spends about five years of his life, or one month each year, doing nothing but waiting.

Here are ten tips he offers for coping with the stress of waiting:

● Go shopping less often. Stock up when you go to the grocery store, so you won't have to waste time waiting on checkout lines.

● Drive less. Avoid frustrating traffic jams by walking, riding a bicycle or using public transportation.

● Phone ahead. Call a store to make sure that what you want is going to be available.

● Shop during off-hours. Avoid crowded stores by shopping during the week or in the evening.

● Read, knit or sew. Having something to do can soothe the nerves during a long wait.

● Educate yourself. Listen to educational tapes on a miniature recorder with an earplug or headset.

● Take a catnap. A snooze is a good way to get through a long wait.

● Shop by mail. You can buy just about anything through a mail-order catalog.

● Christmas shop all year long. Don't wait for the busy holiday season. When you find a good Christmas gift, buy it.

● Write a letter. If you expect a long wait at someone's office, bring pen and paper. Writing a letter helps make time fly.

Ted and Cindy are waiting in line in the discount drugstore. Cindy is picking up some film before she returns to the office after lunch with a friend. Ted is just starting out on his lunch break, and he's using the whole hour for chores.

Cindy is getting more and more impatient, and, as the woman at the front of the line starts to argue with the sales clerk about getting a cash refund for the item she is returning, Cindy breaks out in a sweat. She starts muttering to herself: "This place is totally mismanaged. There should be a special line for returning merchandise. There aren't enough clerks to handle the lunchtime crowds. My boss should do his own chores, I'm not his servant."

Ted is standing directly behind Cindy, but he isn't listening as she goes through her list of complaints. He's into the last thirty pages of a terrific book. Ted figured that he might run into some crowds as he did his chores, so he brought some reading material along.

Finally, Cindy explodes. She walks to the front of the line and shoves her receipt for her boss's film at the sales clerk saying, "This is the last time I come to this store. You shouldn't be running an operation like this if you can't afford to hire the help you need. Well, you've lost my business. I've got more important things to do than stand in line all day!"

Cindy has created her own dilemma. Knowing how crowded the stores are at lunch, she should have left more time to complete her errand. She could have stopped in before lunch and picked up the film. Or, she could have had a shorter meal with her friend and left enough time for the inevitable wait in line. If she had brought a magazine to skim while in line, the whole experience wouldn't have gotten the best of her.

Waiting in lines of one sort or another is one of the most common stress-makers. Next time you're trapped in a slow-moving line, try these tips prepared from advice by Dr. James R. Richmond, senior psychiatrist with the Tulare County Mental Health Services in California; Dr. Dan O'Banion, former joint director of the Institute of Health Psychology at North Texas State University; and Dr. Alan Gruber, director of behavioral medicine, South Shore Counseling Associates, Hanover, Massachusetts.

1. Carry a miniature radio or tape recorder with you and listen to music or an interesting talk show while you're waiting.

2. Chat with others in the line. Make a joke about the

long wait, like, "It has to be worse than this in Russia." If you're in line at an amusement park, ask other people where they're from or what attractions they've tried and enjoyed.

3. If the long line is a result of mismanagement, use the time to mentally compose a letter or phone call to the operator of the place, pointing out politely how he could eliminate the bottleneck.

4. When trapped in a line at the airport, relieve the tedium by helping an older person or a woman traveling alone with their baggage. As soon as you stop focusing on yourself, your impatience will vanish.

5. Carry a puzzle in your pocket, or a miniature game or quiz book. With your mind occupied, you'll find yourself at the front of the line in no time at all.

6. In a line at a restaurant, ask for a copy of the menu, so you can choose what you're going to have ahead of time. Think how much you're going to enjoy the meal. Tell yourself the wait is worth it, or you wouldn't be there in the first place.

7. Try people watching. Observing others can be fun and fascinating. Try to imagine what their lives might be like, as a novelist might do.

TIPS TO RELIEVE TRAFFIC JAM FRUSTRATION

You're late for an important appointment—and you get caught in a traffic jam. You become tense, frustrated and angry. Sound familiar? Next time you get hung up in traffic or stopped at the tracks by a never-ending train, follow these tips from Dr. Robert Amstadter, a psychiatrist and the medical director of the Sacred Heart Lodge Hospital in El Monte, California.

Scream. With your car windows rolled up so no one can hear you, let loose by simple screaming. This releases anxiety.

Snack. Keep a bag of munchies in the glove compartment just for such emergencies. Snacks help take your mind off the traffic and reduce your tension.

Play the radio. Turn on your car radio, and, if it's already on, turn up the volume or switch to another station.

Flex your stomach. Inhale with a deep breath. Gradually, exhale a series of short breaths through your mouth. Next, hold your breath with your stomach in, keeping it taut for a few seconds. *(Don't do this right after eating, or if you have a heart condition.)*

Do isometric exercises. Tense different muscles of the body for a few moments, then relax them. This substitutes muscular tension for psychological tension. *(Don't do this, if you have a heart condition.)*

Do neck turns. If your car isn't moving, gradually rotate your head from left to right in a circle and back again. Repeat as time allows and you'll feel more relaxed.

Stretch your back. If you get a chance, sit upright, bend your elbows and raise them shoulder level with your fists clenched tightly. Next, take a deep breath, then thrust your elbows back forcefully while you exhale.

Exercise your ankles. Press the ball of one foot against the floorboard and rotate the ankle from left to right and back again. Do the same for your other ankle. Repeat as time allows.

"Every one of these exercises helps break the concentration on whatever is making you tense," says Dr. Amstadter.

AVOIDING CHRISTMAS-RUSH TENSION

Christmas shopping can be a real hassle—the rush, the crowds, the harried salesclerks. But there are ways to take the stress out of holiday gift buying, say two experts.

Here are the suggestions of Dr. Anthony Pietropinto, a New York psychiatrist, and Dr. William Mindak, a Tulane University professor of marketing, to make your Christmas shopping stress-free:

If you shop on a cold, windy, rainy or snowy day, "stores generally are less crowded," says Dr. Pietropinto. "Parking spaces are more plentiful and sales assistants are not so busy."

Don't shop when you're not in the mood. "If you wake up feeling a little grouchy, tired or with a headache, put off your shopping trip until you feel better," Dr. Pietropinto advises.

Try to shop early in the week. Some stores do up to 70 percent of their business on Thursday, Friday and Saturday, Dr. Mindak points out. Do your Christmas buying on a Monday or Tuesday, since these are traditionally slow days in the retail business.

If possible, don't shop with small children. "Why complicate things? Children asking for goodies or asking to go to rest rooms—not to mention getting lost—can make your shopping twice as worrisome," says Dr. Mindak.

Avoid wasting time and energy when you shop. Instead of running up and down from floor to floor in a department store, start at the top floor, where it's generally less crowded, and work your way down.

Plan your shopping in advance. Use newspaper advertisements to help you decide what to buy and where to buy it. If you're buying clothes, jot down everybody's size before you go shopping.

Keep all your sales slips in a file folder. You may need them later, if gifts have to be exchanged or returned for a refund. "Lose those slips and you can be sure of a stress-filled encounter with store management," warns Dr. Pietropinto, medical director of the mental health program at Lutheran Medical Center in Brooklyn.

Finally, make Christmas shopping fun. Look at the ornaments and decorations. Play with toys. Pause to watch Santa talking to the children. Listen to the carols being played on the store loudspeakers. Treat yourself to lunch. By putting yourself in the Christmas spirit, you'll have a good time.

ROCK MUSIC CAN BE HAZARDOUS TO YOUR HEALTH

Listening to a certain type of rock music raises stress and, therefore, increases your susceptibility to disease, says Dr. John Diamond, a New York psychiatrist. "I'm not saying rock music causes cancer or anything like that," he explains. "But it weakens the body and raises your vulnerability to whatever [illness] is going around."

Dr. Diamond, who is past president of the International Academy of Preventive Medicine, said he tested more than twenty thousand recordings before he learned that certain rock tempos throw the heart out of synchronization. "The beat started with the Supremes in about 1965," he explained. "What this beat sounds like is dit-dit-da, dit-dit-da. It not only has the accent on the third beat, it has the psychological effect of stoppage. In other words, it's the opposite of the beat of the heart.

"When we tape record the sound of the heart and blood vessels, the heart is going 'da-dit' and the blood vessels are going 'da-dit-dit, da-dit-dit.' Both of these are the opposite of the beat in rock.

"What we suspect is happening is that we constantly monitor our heartbeat and, when we hear this rock beat, we subconsciously say, 'Something has gone wrong with the heart,' and a stress signal is set up. And in this stress condition, we lose life energy."

Dr. Diamond, former professor of psychiatry at New York's Mt. Sinai School of Medicine, said this "dit-dit-da" beat could be found in music by the Bee Gees, Janis Joplin, Jimi Hendrix, Rod Stewart, the Rolling Stones, Paul McCartney's Wings group and others.

Ironically, he said, the harmful beat is not found in disco and punk rock music, nor is it in any of Elvis Presley's music. He added that it is never found in music by the great composers, such as Bach, Beethoven, Brahms and others, nor is it in waltzes or "easy-listening" music.

"Music is one of the great therapies," he concluded. "Anytime you're not feeling right, play some music. It can really have an effect on your life." Just be certain you choose the kind of sound that strengthens your body, rather than weakens it.

STRESS AND THE DAILY NEWS—HOW TO DODGE IT

If a daily dose of bad news is getting you down, take a vacation from it and you'll feel like a vibrant new person. "Much of what we call 'news' is not new at all," says Dr. Fredrick Koenig, professor of social psychology at Tulane University. "The stories are simply beefed up from day to day with new wrinkles."

Dr. Emery Breitner, a psychiatrist and director of

the Institute for Group Dynamics in Roslyn, New York, adds: "Following the news so closely, in fact, is extremely anxiety provoking. It makes us suspicious, guarded and even frightened."

Here's what you can do: kick the news habit. By doing this, Dr. Breitner says "you'll relieve tension, add a sunny disposition to your life and find time for the really important things you didn't think you had time to do." You can still remain well-informed and significantly reduce stress, according to Dr. Koenig, simply by reading a news magazine or week-in-review section every weekend.

Dr. Koenig suggests that spouses take turns reading or watching the news. More time could be spent talking with your neighbors and catching up with what's going on in the community. You can also spend more time with your family.

By cutting down on news, "you'll have a much more peaceful week and find that not much has changed," Dr. Breitner concludes.

LOUD NOISE CAN BE A KILLER

Loud noise and related influences, such as vibrations or flashing lights, created stress that depletes the body's supply of magnesium and increases your risk of heart attack, experts say.

"High decibel sounds that bombard us through the day can rob us of magnesium and increase our risk of heart disease," declares Dr. Carl Johnson, an environmental health expert. "Magnesium deficiency can cause blood vessels to the heart to constrict and go into spasm. This cuts off the supply of blood to the heart, leading to a heart attack."

Dr. Mildred Seelig, associate professor of clinical

medicine at New York University, agrees, pointing out that a magnesium deficiency leaves excess calcium in the heart, which can also trigger heart attacks by causing irregular heartbeats, as well as clotting and blocking of arteries.

Studies made in West Germany clearly show the harmful effects of loud noise. In one experiment twelve men were examined after working five days in a noisy brewery, where the sound level was about 95 decibels. Then they were reexamined after working five days with earplugs which reduced the noise level to 82 decibels. The magnesium level in their red blood cells was 5 percent lower on the noisy days, according to Dr. Hartmut Ising, Ph.D., the physicist who made the studies.

In a second experiment, forty-five people worked one day with the taped sound of loud traffic blasting from a loudspeaker. The next day, they worked with only routine background sounds around them. Their red cell magnesium level was 1.5 percent lower on the noisy day, Dr. Ising reported.

Experts say you can help protect yourself from the stressful effects of noise in the following ways:

You should eat foods which are rich in magnesium—fish, shellfish, leafy greens, beans, vegetables, whole grains, nuts. Cut down on red meats and dairy products. Be aware that processed foods lose some of their magnesium due to additives. And take a magnesium supplement. The recommended dose is about 250 milligrams daily.

You can also avoid water softeners; these substitute sodium for magnesium.

Listen to "quiet" music, instead of listening to loud rock music. Develop a taste for music with quieter tones, such as classical music. Avoid loud sounds whenever possible. Stay away from construction sites, from noisy clubs where loud music is played, noisy lunchrooms, etc. Shut out noise by closing the windows of your home or office when garbage trucks are working outside or when a neighbor is using a power lawn mower. Use earplugs when you use a hair dryer or if you're working in noisy surroundings.

Or move away from noise. If a noisy washing machine or dishwasher or air conditioner is running in your home, if someone is playing the radio or television at high volume, move to another room. By giving yourself periods of quiet, you give your body the opportunity to renew its magnesium supply.

CHAPTER IV

Quick and Easy Stress Relievers for Everyday Life

MENTAL RELAXATION TECHNIQUES, ACUPRESSURE, EXercises and nutrition can all help to protect you from stress. How about daydreaming, sighing, groaning and laughing your way to better health? If you're in the office, driving a truck, having a fight with the store manager, you may not have the time or composure to analyze exactly what's bugging you and the best way to handle it. A good laugh might just do the trick. If you're sitting in the car, hung up in gridlock, maybe a wiggle of your toes or relaxing your jaw will bring you some relief. Most of us could benefit by building some quick stress-relievers into our day. Let's have a look at some popular remedies.

The "Quick-Charge" Method of Relaxation

You can deal more effectively with stress if you use the "quick-charge" technique for relaxing. It can be mastered in minutes, says Dr. Deborah Bright, adjunct professor of education at Wayne State University, Detroit.

The quick-charge method gives you a burst of needed energy for handling those stomach-knotting, chest-tightening moments when you're face-to-face with stress.

"It's like giving a run-down battery a quick charge, and it's proved to be amazingly successful. You cannot avoid stress and you can't eliminate the stressor. But you can change your reactions to stressful situations by the quick-charge method," explains Dr. Bright.

The first step is to learn to recognize your own stress symptoms. They could be a headache, a knot in the stomach, tightening of the chest, sweaty, clammy palms, clenching of the jaws, flushing of the face, erratic breathing or a change in your tone of voice.

When you realize you're getting tense, stop whatever you're doing and give yourself a quick-charge. "Start by inhaling deeply," says Dr. Bright, "then exhaling slowly and smoothly. Disguise it as a sigh, if you like. A sigh is quite acceptable in our society, and it will start to relax you."

Here are some sample stress-producing situations and specific examples of quick-charge techniques.

SITUATION: Your child spills milk all over the kitchen floor you've just spent a half hour cleaning.

QUICK-CHARGE: "Begin to breathe deeply," suggests Dr. Bright. "Say to yourself: 'So what! So what if life isn't going exactly the way I want it to go. It's not such a big deal.' Ask yourself: 'What am I going to do about it?' You'll be realizing already that getting angry isn't going to clean up the milk. Then clean up the mess and quickly forget about it."

SITUATION: The electric range isn't working and the repairman who promised to be there at 10 A.M. hasn't arrived by 3 P.M.

QUICK-CHARGE: "Give yourself permission to feel sorry for yourself for exactly three minutes—no more. Cuss and complain and gripe about the problem for three minutes—and then get on with something else. The unwanted stress is gone."

SITUATION: Your boss calls you in and criticizes your work.

QUICK-CHARGE: "As soon as you feel your stress level rising, stop talking. That is crucial. Light a cigarette, blow your nose, cough—anything to give you time to think. Inhale and exhale deeply, thinking of what you want to say. Use the time while your boss is talking to get in touch with yourself. Then reply calmly and slowly. You'll have saved yourself unnecessary stress— and perhaps your job."

SITUATION: You get into an argument with your neighbor, who's making a silly complaint. You can get as angry as he is and risk escalating the argument into a fist-fight. Or . . .

QUICK-CHARGE: "Look straight at him—and picture him as an ostrich, a laughing hyena or a penguin. Suddenly, you'll get everything into perspective and stop taking a petty situation seriously. And he'll never guess what he said to make you smile so happily!"

Dr. Bright also makes the following general recommendations:

"Take an inventory of the issues that are causing you anxiety. Rate them like money. Are they five-cent issues or dollar issues? Most of them, you'll realize, are worth just a nickel, and definitely not worth worrying about. It's like the couple who are going out to dinner with friends. The wife has taken down the directions, and they get lost. Her husband reacts by shouting at her. His stress level rises, so does hers—and it doesn't get them where they're going. If he'd stopped to think, he would have realized that he was hurting the one he loved and ruining the evening—all for a five-cent argument.

"One of the most stressful things that can happen is a husband or wife dumping the frustrations of the day on their spouse. Suddenly, they're two explosive human beings. Instead, use a quick-charge technique to avoid an explosion. Before you meet, rate your mood on a one-to-ten stress scale. If you've had a rotten day, the score will be over five, and you don't talk about it.

"Often the first sign of approaching stress is a knot in the stomach. When it happens, breathe in deeply, clench your stomach muscles. Exhale slowly, relaxing the stomach muscles, and imagine your tummy getting a coating of thick, pink, smooth Pepto-Bismol. Repeat several times if necessary. You'll be astonished at how quickly that rush of anxiety will subside.

"Determine exactly what you want. One of my clients was a working wife who got home one night and told her husband she wanted to eat out. He agreed, and took her for a hamburger. But what she really meant was that she wanted a romantic, candlelit dinner. If you determine specifically what you want, you increase your chances of being satisfied at the end.

"When things are really getting on top of you, don't try to forget your worries. Just gather them all up together in your mind and imagine making a tape recording of them all. Then picture yourself putting the cassette on a tape recorder—and pressing the erase button.

"When your problems seem worst, apply this test: will this be something I'm still worried about in a year's time? Suddenly, you'll realize how small the problem really is."

Wiping Worries Away
with the
"Spot Technique"

Get rid of your worries with an incredibly simple "spot technique," says Dr. Herbert Hoffman, director of the Hillside Psychological Guidance Center in Queens Village, New York. "It's a way to let your mind go blank. The spot technique helps clear your mind and banish all disturbing thoughts."

Here's how the method works:

Find a quiet spot where you won't be disturbed. Once you are comfortable, "tell yourself that, when your 'spot' session is over, you'll have peace of mind, feel refreshed and anxiety-free," says Dr. Hoffman.

Now close your eyes and focus your attention on an imaginary spot in the center of your forehead. Picture the spot as clearly as you can in your mind. If you have a problem imagining the spot, Hoffman suggests you press your forefinger to your brow or moisten a dime and then press it into place so "it will stick to your forehead and give you something more tangible to focus on."

Mentally make the spot disappear. Imagine it getting smaller and smaller, until it finally vanishes. "When it's gone—or is as small as you can make it—your 'spot' session is over," Dr. Hoffman explains. "Open your eyes and you'll find your mind free of disturbing thoughts for up to a half hour."

Use the technique once or twice a day. With practice you should eventually be able to "blank" your mind in less than ten seconds.

Knowing the Right
Word Can
Cut Anxiety

By choosing a "special" word that makes you feel good—and repeating it twice a day for a few minutes at a time—you can reduce stress and improve your general health, according to Dr. M. Lawrence Furst, a research psychologist at Philadelphia's Temple University.

Dr. Furst, an associate professor of behavioral sciences at Temple, co-conducted a four-year university study, which showed that repeating a word which arouses your positive feelings can cut stress and anxiety. In explaining the simple technique, Dr. Furst advises finding the single word that works best for you, because the ideal word varies from person to person.

"First, think of a situation where you normally feel very relaxed. It might be taking a bath, being in the mountains, soaking up sun on the beach, reading a book or watching your favorite TV show. If, for example, it's the beach that attracts you most, select a number of words that might give you the images of the beach. Think of words like 'sea,' 'water,' 'sand,' 'sky,' 'sun,' 'wave.' You can even use the word 'beach,' if it works for you.

"Then close your eyes for a moment and say each of the words to yourself five times. Find the one that gives you the most pleasant image. That's your special word.

"Now find a place where you're comfortable—in a chair or on a couch. Make sure the TV is off and the lights are low. Sit down, close your eyes and repeat your word to yourself—at your own pace—for about five minutes. Don't lie down, because you might fall asleep.

"Now your mind is at the beach. You feel very relaxed. Your breathing and heart rate have slowed down. Try to do this twice a day, before breakfast and dinner. The more you practice, the easier it will be."

Dr. Furst says that this technique, which can be mastered in seven to ten days, can be used in a number of ways.

● "Use it before you drive home through heavy traffic.

● "If you're a woman coping with children all day, take a five-minute break with the technique.

● "I use this technique to help people give up smoking. Instead of going for a cigarette, take a five-minute meditation break. At the end, suggest to yourself: 'I don't need that cigarette now. I feel fine.'

● "If you're dieting, the minute you get an urge to eat between meals, take a minibreak and use the word technique. Then say to yourself: 'I'm going to feel full. I won't need to cheat on my diet.'"

The Temple University study tested the technique on seventy-two men and women of various ages. None of the participants suffered from any extreme personality disorders, but some were highly stressed individuals. With a ninety-six-page questionnaire, such factors as stress, anxiety, fatigue and depression were measured, before and after the meditation.

"There's no question the subjects had temporary benefits, which were shown by reduced pulse and breathing rates," Dr. Furst reported. "Over the long term, I'm convinced they'll have such things as lower blood pressure."

Laugh for Your Health

Having a good giggle can do more for you than you think. Humor can make you more productive and efficient by reducing stress. And it is possible to learn how to laugh at life's problems, experts say.

"Humor is an important coping tool," explains Dr. Vera Robinson, author of *Humor and the Health Professions*. "It's a healthy release for the anxiety and tension that build up in everyday life and hold people back from their best performance."

One recent study showed that students who were told jokes before a test scored significantly higher on the test than students who weren't told jokes. Another study found that people who work in environments where humor is encouraged showed more enthusiasm for their jobs.

Dr. William Fry, a Stanford University psychiatrist, has been studying the beneficial effects of laughter for twenty-five years. He is coauthor of *Make 'Em Laugh* and says that laughing not only increases the heartbeat rate, giving the heart a good workout, but "it's a good exercise for the rest of your body, too—the muscles in your chest, abdomen, diaphragm, face, neck and sometimes your arms and legs, when you're laughing really hard. And, after this exercise experience, your muscles become relaxed and you become less tense. A Harvard study of successful and fulfilled people found that humor was one of the major coping mechanisms they used to deal with the challenges and stresses."

Here's what you can do to develop your sense of humor:

1. See what makes people around you laugh. The

next time you're on a bus or in a store, listen to how often people laugh and what they find funny.

2. Start your own humor library. Collect books that amuse you and cut out funny cartoons. Then look through your collection regularly to help you develop a responsiveness to humor.

3. Flip to the cartoon section of the newspaper, after you've read the front page. This will give you a humorous perspective on world events and remind you that life isn't as serious as we all think.

4. Watch television comedy shows. Try to discover the message these programs offer—that we can laugh in the face of difficulty.

"Humor isn't trivial and superficial," insists Dr. Fry. "It's an important part of all human activity."

Dr. Robinson adds: "When you laugh, you let go of anger, frustration, anxiety and hostility. That frees a person's energy so he can do more of whatever job he has to do."

Speaking of Gossip . . .
It's Good for You

Imagine! One of our favorite pastimes has hidden virtues. If you enjoy a good gossip session around the water cooler or over the back fence, stop feeling guilty and go right ahead. Gossip can relieve stress, help you share your opinions, and ease the way to meeting new people.

"Gossip actually lets people express their outrage, anger and also irritation at other people's behavior," explains Dr. John Sabini, associate professor of psychology at the University of Pennsylvania. And gossiping about someone else can help you find out whether or not your friends and coworkers actually share your opinions, he adds. "Most people find it reassuring and also comforting when their views are shared by everyone else. For example, if someone you know is having an affair, it can easily be discussed with gossip, letting people approve or disapprove."

Through gossip, you can also meet and become acquainted with new people. "If you're at a bus stop, in a dentist's waiting room or even at the office coffee machine, gossip is a good way to break the ice," suggests Dr. Sabini. "You can talk about a well-known celebrity, a local personality, a coworker.

"And gossip can also be fun. It's a kind of entertainment that people can enjoy for free at home."

Go Ahead and Reminisce—It Can Add Years to Your Life

Remember when you were little and Christmas was sheer ecstasy? Or the thrill of getting your first car? Or the joy of the birth of your first child? Go ahead—remember. It's good for you. Recalling the happy times in your past can reduce stress, give you more joy, ease the pain of current disappointments—and add years to your life.

"Reminiscing serves an important mental function," reports Dr. Pietro Castelnuovo-Tedesco, professor of psychiatry at Vanderbilt University School of Medicine in Nashville, Tennessee. "It helps you stay in touch with yourself and with previous editions of yourself.

"Studies by psychologists at retirement homes show that old people who reminisce freely and more openly tend to live longer than residents who don't," said Dr. Castelnuovo-Tedesco. "Reminiscing put more joy into their existence and protected them more against disappointments in the present." Three such studies concluded that "reminiscing reduces not only stress, but illness and ailments of all types."

The benefits of reminiscing aren't confined to the elderly, either, he adds. "Everybody reminisces—but many people feel a little guilty about it or feel they're wasting time. Those who try to block normal reminiscing probably pay a penalty, because they have less sense of contact with themselves. You get strength from reminding yourself that you've changed in some ways, but not in others.

"If you think of how you were as a sophomore in high school, you'll think of yourself as being older now, but more mature, more experienced, more capable. So you have a sense of growth and development. But in other essential things, such as liking and disliking some types of people, you haven't changed. So we also get a sense of strength from knowing that we're still the same person we were.

"And we use memories to restore ourselves. We feed on our good memories, especially when things aren't going so well in our present lives. If you're fired, for example, it's good for you to reminisce about more successful times." Or, if you're having trouble with a teenage child, a live-in, elderly parent or a cantankerous spouse, think back to the way it was. It can be the great escape.

Take a Daydream Vacation and Beat the Blues

"Step right up! Step right up and get two tickets to the vacation of a lifetime!" It's a dream of a deal and it's all yours, all expenses paid. Dream is the operative word here. Pleasant fantasies—simple daydreams—can reduce stress and relieve everyday anxieties.

A "fantasy vacation" can be a particularly good way to banish tension, say psychologists Dr. Robert Fleer and Dr. Stephen Thayer. Here's how to take an armchair vacation to your Fantasy Island:

Decide where you want to go—a tropical island, the bright lights of Las Vegas. "Maybe you'd just like to get back to a lake where you spent some time in the summer, or to a mountain resort you visited last winter," Dr. Thayer suggests.

Prepare in advance for your "trip" by picking up a few travel brochures or a travel book at the library. Read about the place you want to visit, so you'll have more to enjoy. Then, sit back in a comfortable place with no distractions. Breathe deeply for a minute or two and get totally relaxed. Play some soft music or perhaps the music of the locale or country you plan to visit, says Dr. Fleer.

Decide if you're taking this vacation alone or with other people. "For some, a fantasy vacation is to get away from everything and leave everyone behind," Dr. Thayer points out. "You might want to go off alone to explore a new city, a new culture or a new world."

Or you might want to take along a friend or a romantic partner—Robert Redford if you're a woman or Brooke Shields if you're a man. "For a lot of people, thinking about romance, whether with someone real or imaginary, is a very pleasant experience.

"Don't feel guilty about this kind of fantasizing, because nobody knows it but you. So let yourself go," advises Dr. Thayer.

Think about packing your bags and choosing which clothes you'll take along. Imagine how you will travel—by jet, luxury liner or limousine. Don't worry about the cost. Go first class all the way. In your fantasy, pretend you have the financial resources to go and the time to do it, Dr. Thayer advises.

Visualize the exotic foods you'll eat during your dream vacation. Imagine the activities you'll enjoy—for example, surfing in Hawaii or watching the headliners perform in Las Vegas. And don't allow any pressures to disrupt your fantasy vacation. If there isn't time to complete your holiday in one sitting, take it in segments. For example, start your vacation in the morning, then continue it later in the evening, when you have more time.

Don't let negative thoughts intrude and spoil your vacation. Forget about your cares and leave your troubles behind. Says Dr. Thayer: "You will feel the benefits, if you let yourself have even ten minutes of fantasy."

Goof Off Sometimes—Procrastination Is an Important Safety Valve

"Never put off until tomorrow what you can do today" is a bit of folk wisdom most of us have been raised on and maybe have even suffered from. There are times when procrastination—putting some things off for another day—can be good for you.

"Procrastination can be used as a tool to help you maintain your mental health and physical well-being," says Dr. Neal Olshan, psychologist and director of the Pain Rehabilitation Center at Mesa Lutheran Hospital in Mesa, Arizona. Procrastination can act as a safety valve in today's stress-filled world. People often take on too many tasks, putting themselves under heavy stress, which can cause serious illness, Dr. Olshan explains. But by putting off some of our tasks, we can relieve the stress and stay healthier in the process.

Procrastination offers another benefit: it helps you determine which tasks are really important and which can easily be put off until later.

"A third way creative procrastination can be good for you is in helping you determine the best and most effective way to accomplish a task," says the psychologist. When you put off a troublesome job until later, it gives your subconscious mind a chance to solve the problem in a better way.

However, Dr. Olshan warns, you should never procrastinate on anything that affects your health or safety. For example, if you have warning symptoms of illness, don't put off seeing a doctor. Or, if your car needs tires, don't postpone getting them.

Sigh Your Troubles Away

"Sigh therapy"—simple breathing exercises—may help you to overcome stress and the bad habits that come with it.

"Many bad habits, such as overeating, smoking, drinking and the misuse of prescription drugs, are reactions to tension and frustration," says psychologist Dr. Alfred Barrios. "Reducing your level of tension can help you reduce your need for these excesses." And reducing tension can be as simple as taking a deep breath and sighing.

"Breathing is one of the easiest and quickest ways of changing the physiology of the body and the psychology of the mind," asserts Dr. Edward Stainbrook, former chairman of the psychiatry department at the University of Southern California School of Medicine. Many people use "sigh therapy" to control stress without even being aware of it. For instance, basketball players and marksmen find that the act of expelling breath just before shooting has a steadying and calming effect.

Breathing techniques have been used as a therapeutic tool in Yoga for centuries. Even smokers will unconsciously use "sigh therapy" each time they light up. "When smokers inhale, they take a deep breath, so breathing is part of the relaxation technique they're already using," says Dr. Stainbrook. "But you don't have to smoke to use this technique. Simply take a deep breath without smoking and you will achieve the same results."

The next time you are about to reach for a cigarette, drink or unnecessary snack, you can use sigh therapy instead. Here are two breathing exercises from Dr. Barrios:

1. Sit down in a comfortable chair, with your arms at your side or resting on the arms of the chair. Take a deep breath, hold it for a count of ten, then exhale or sigh, letting your breath out all at once and allowing your body to go completely loose and limp. Repeat at one-minute intervals until you feel more relaxed.

2. While breathing normally, relax as you exhale. Count slowly from twenty down to ten, one number per breath. With every breath that you take, try to relax even more. Since this technique involves normal breathing, it can be done anywhere and any time.

Groan . . . You'll Feel Better

Gggrrrr! Aaarrgghhh! That's right. Everyone all together now Aaaaawwwwwhhh! You've got it—groaning. Let's give one groan for washing the car, two groans for cooking dinner, three groans for doing your homework and ten groans for doing your income taxes. Now how do you feel? Better? Well, it will come as no surprise to Dr. Louis M. Savary, coauthor of a book on stress. Dr. Savary says a simple groan is "an instant, guaranteed stress-reliever. It provides a healthy way to deal with pain, and it provides immediate, temporary relief for certain emotional pressures and stresses."

Dr. Savary, adjunct professor at Sacred Heart University in Bridgeport, Connecticut, says that groaning, without being overly strenuous or time-consuming, helps a person physically relax. "And physical relaxation is one of the most essential needs of people under any severe stress." When a person groans, he explains, the entire body is involved in a "gentle, rhythmic activity which requires deep and regulated breathing. This supplies maximum amounts of oxygen to all parts of the body.

"Groaning also provides psychological relief, for it focuses attention away from what ails you. I usually suggest that 'groaners' imaginatively picture their anger, hurt, fear or frustration, and visualize these tension-producing feelings being released from their bodies with every exhaled breath and groan.

"Anyone who's ever attended a sporting event has experienced this sensation, for it's the one place where groaning is totally acceptable. When the hometown football team misses a touchdown pass or the star batter strikes out or the local basketball favorite fails to score on a free throw, the entire stadium erupts in a mass groan. You can hear the entire audience grieve in unison, as everyone relieves their stress in an ear-splitting sound.

"Groaning is also a form of psychological self-comfort. It's a way of showing yourself compassion. Often it's very healthy to feel sorry for yourself, for this allows you to express and acknowledge your emotional pain, instead of denying those feelings and keeping them bottled up inside, where they may eventually cause you more suffering. When you bury your hurts, they are apt to erupt when you least expect them to—as the trigger of a psychosomatic ailment or an obstruction to an honest relationship with someone close."

Here is Dr. Savary's basic formula for getting instant relief from physical and emotional stress:

"Just stop what you are doing and groan deeply for at least ten minutes. Either lie down or sit perfectly straight, so the spine is erect. You want to be in a position where your windpipe is not bent, so that the air flow is unobstructed and complete. If you're humped over, the groan will be strained and you'll be hampered from making the proper sounds.

"A good groan begins with a deep breath that distends and seems to fill the lower intestines. The pressure felt there and then pushed out meets momentary resistance in the throat, where the sound of the groan begins. When the throat is fully opened, the contained air rushes out, and as it passes the voice box, creates the sound we usually associate with groaning—a long, grieving expression of meaningless vowel sounds.

"Give yourself permission to make lots of noise, to get those sounds out and not be embarrassed by the experience. Clearly, it may be advisable to warn your family what you're doing, so they don't rush to call the doctor or an emergency service. If you cannot arrange your groaning sessions at a time when you're alone in the house, you might turn on the radio loud enough to muffle the sounds or do your groaning while in the shower.

"To get the full calming effects out of a groaning session, invest your groans with all the emotions you can generate by using your imagination to visualize all the sources of your angers and frustration. For example, if your kids have been driving you up the wall, think of how much you'd like to take a swat at them—and groan. If it's your boss, your mate or the repairmen who never come on time when you need them, groan out your feelings with all the intensity you can muster. Have specific targets for your groans. Let out all those built-up feelings which haven't had any place to go.

"After just a few minutes of groaning, you'll find your groans are naturally becoming quieter and developing into a moan or a sigh. That's a sign that you've rid yourself of accumulated tension—the body's signal that you've experienced relief, because the excess pressure is released, the tension is gone and the anxiety is over."

You can do your groaning regularly, at set times or whenever the mood moves you, Dr. Savary says. Five or ten minutes is usually sufficient to give relief. "If you do it longer, you're apt to strain your throat," he cautions.

Hobbies as Therapy . . .
They Can Literally Save Lives

"Only about 25 percent of Americans actually enjoy the work they do to make a living," says psychologist

Dr. Samuel Janus, professor at New York Medical College. "All of these [other] people could use some satisfaction that their jobs don't provide. A creative hobby can fill that gap. As they see something actually take shape at their hands, they feel a great sense of self-worth."

Take the case of George L. At forty-three, he was a prime candidate for ulcers and alcoholism because of on-the-job stress. He told his wife, "I feel as though I'm in a vise." His escape was to stop at a neighborhood bar on the way home from work. But George soon found that he needed more and more alcohol to relax.

Then one day he met an artist in the bar and marveled at the man's composure and easygoing attitude toward life. On the way home, George bought some paints and canvas. The next night, instead of stopping at the bar, he went straight home to paint.

Since that new beginning, George has given up alcohol for painting. For an hour each evening, he immerses himself completely in his hobby. He leaves his work worries at the plant and is a happier and more energetic man.

Dr. Donald Dudley, psychiatrist and professor at the University of Washington in Seattle, adds: "A hobby is more than a good idea. In our culture it's a necessity. And from the standpoint of the usual American, who plans to work a certain number of years and then retire, hobbies literally save lives. We are pretty high-geared people, and, if you maintain a very high-energy output for a lot of years, then suddenly stop, you can almost guarantee that you're going to get a stroke or heart attack."

The Physical Side of Stress Relief

Maybe your problems are too serious to laugh at. Or perhaps your memories are too painful and you find daydreaming a waste of time. Whatever the reason, exercises and techniques of a physical nature just might appeal to you more than mental exercises. It doesn't matter. You should use any and all means—if they are safe, healthy and legal—to get some relief from stress, if it's dragging you down. Who knows? The harder you try and the more you experiment with stress relief based on the many ideas in this book, the closer you may come to tailoring your own program for your own needs.

DO-IT-YOURSELF ACUPRESSURE

If you have a headache that just won't quit and you feel like banging your head against the wall—don't. Help is just around the corner. You can ease the damaging stress brought on by tension, anxiety and depression, as well as relieve yourself of a wide variety of everyday aches and pains, by using acupressure. All you have to do is press firmly with your finger on the correct body point, says acupressure specialist Dr. Robert E. Willner.

There are twenty-five body points commonly used in acupressure. Figures 1, 2 and 3 give the location of twenty-two of these points.

Dr. Willner, who is the author of three books about acupressure, recommends that you sit or lie down during the treatment, which is relaxing and may make you sleepy. Use one of these two methods: a) apply

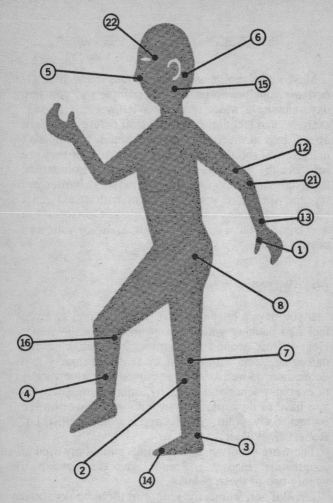

Figure 1

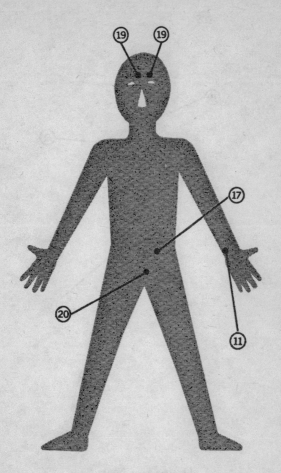

Figure 2 — front

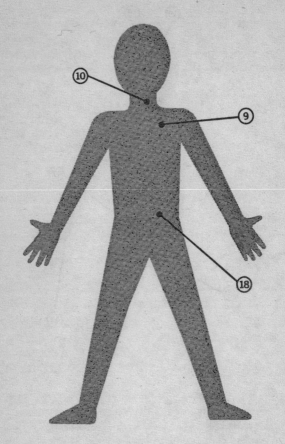

Figure 3 — back

pressure to the appropriate point, until you feel mild discomfort, and continue the pressure for a period of about one to two minutes, or b) press firmly for a slow count of ten, release for a count of ten, press again and continue doing this three to six times. Use either method several times a day, as necessary.

CAUTION: Many of the ailments listed are also symptomatic of illnesses. You should always check with your doctor (or psychiatrist, in the case of anxiety, tension, or depression) before using acupressure.

DON'TS: AVOID treatment after eating.
DO NOT use acupressure if you are pregnant.
DO NOT use acupressure if you are a heart patient.
DO NOT apply acupressure to inflamed areas of the skin, or where a rash, scar or infection is present.

INSTRUCTIONS: The following list shows which acupressure points to use for some specific problems. Before you begin the treatment, make sure you have clean fingers and well-trimmed nails to avoid injury or infection.

Locate the correct area on your body and press it with the ball of your finger. "It will feel like a gnawing pain when you hit it," Dr. Willner points out. "When more than one point is indicated for an ailment, use all of them."

Allergy: point 5
Anxiety: 1, 11 and 13
Arm pain: 9, 12 and 21

Back pain: 3, 6 and 18
Constipation: 2 and 17
Depression: 1, 10, 11 and 13
Diarrhea: 2 and 17
Emotional stress: 1, 11 and 13
Face pain: 1, 14 and 15
Frigidity: 4, 18, and 20
Headaches: 1, 3 and 6, plus point 22 for temple area and point 19 for over the eyes
Impotency: 4, 18 and 20
Indigestion: 2 and 17
Itching: 2 and 16
Jaw pain: 14
Menstrual disorders: 2, 4 and 20
Migraines: 1 and 11
Muscle aches: 7
Nausea: 2, 4 and 16
Neck pain: 1, 6 and 9
Nervousness: 1, 11 and 13
Shoulder pain: 1, 7 and 9
Stomachaches: 2
Tension: 1, 11 and 13

*THE "QUIETING RESPONSE": SIX SECONDS
TO RELIEF*

If you can breathe, you can do this exercise. You don't need strength, energy or even jogging shoes. In fact, you don't even work up a sweat. The revolutionary six-second technique, called the "Quieting Response" (QR), can be done anytime, anywhere and can eliminate emotional stress caused by everyday situations.

"To understand how and why QR works, you need to know how your body reacts to stress," advises the researcher who developed the exercise, Dr. Charles Stroebel. At the first sign of stress, you may feel yourself blush, your palms turn sweaty. Then the muscles of your face tense up and your body temperature drops, causing your hands and feet to feel cold and clammy. Finally, your jaw becomes clenched.

"QR takes all these reactions and reverses them," says Dr. Stroebel. He describes the exercise as follows:

● When tension strikes, relax your facial muscles.

● Smile inwardly. Imagine a smile coming across your face and spreading up to your eyes. "Think to yourself: 'My eyes are twinkling and sparkling.'

● "You should consciously think of calmness and tranquillity, getting your facial muscles out of that grim posture of an angry dog going into battle."

● Take a deep breath and imagine you are inhaling through holes in the bottoms of your feet, up through your legs and into your stomach. "You will experience flowing warmth and heaviness," says Dr. Stroebel.

● Finally, slowly exhale, imagining the air is flowing back down through your legs. Let your jaw, tongue and shoulders go limp.

CAUTION: People taking medication for epilepsy, diabetes or high blood pressure should check with their doctors before they try QR, advises Dr. Stroebel, who is research director of the world-renowned Institute of Living in Hartford, Connecticut. "This is because, if you do QR and you're on medication, you may need the dosage adjusted downward, as QR relieves your stress."

FIFTEEN SIMPLE EXERCISES TO HELP YOU RELAX

Anyone who has ever followed a regular exercise program—faithfully—can offer testimony on the physical and mental benefits. So why not exercises designed to melt away stress? Dr. Alfred Coodley, a University of Southern California medical school psychiatrist, and other experts at the Harvard and Vanderbilt University medical schools have devised just such a program to cut stress.

"These exercises can truly help you cut down stress to safe levels," says Dr. Coodley. "Anybody can do them, regardless of age or physical condition. They can cut your stress in half—without drugs. You do them in logical order, from head to toe. They can be done sitting in a chair or lying on your back. Some can be done anywhere—sitting in your office, at a traffic light or cooking at your stove—and nobody will even know you're exercising."

Try to perform all the exercises twice daily, in the morning and evening. Even if you have time for only a few, they still help reduce stress. During the routine, which takes less than ten minutes, each exercise should be performed once, unless otherwise indicated. Following each exercise, relax for at least ten seconds.

Here are the experts' fifteen steps to greater relaxation:

1. FOREHEAD: Arch your eyebrows as high as you can. Hold them there for ten seconds, then release them suddenly. Relax. Now frown deeply, lowering your eyebrows as far as you can. Hold for ten seconds. Release suddenly. Relax.

2. EYES: Close your eyes tightly. Hold for ten seconds, then flick them open. Relax.

3. NOSE AND CHEEKS: Wrinkle up your nose

and raise your cheeks at the same time. Hold ten seconds. Release quickly. Relax.

4. MOUTH: Press your lips together as tightly as you can. Feel the tendons under your chin getting taut. Hold ten seconds. Release suddenly. Relax.

5. TONGUE: Bring the tip of your tongue up against the roof of your mouth, behind your upper teeth, pressing hard. Muscles around the jaw and under the chin should feel taut. Hold ten seconds, then let go quickly. Relax.

6. NECK: In a high-backed chair or lying down, press your head back. Hold ten seconds, then release quickly. Relax. Or, rotate your head in a circle slowly, first one way, and then the other, two or three times.

7. SHOULDERS: Raise your shoulders in a shrug, as high as you can. At the same time, extend your arms stiffly behind you and angled outward, with your palms facing back and thumbs pointing down. Hold ten seconds, then suddenly drop your shoulders. Relax.

8. CHEST: Slowly draw the deepest breath you can. Hold it for at least six seconds. Exhale quickly. Relax. Do this four times.

9. UPPER ARMS: Touch your fingertips to your shoulder, while tensing your biceps—the big muscles in your upper arms—so they enlarge. Hold tense for ten seconds, then suddenly let go. Relax.

10. LOWER ARMS: Hold your arms straight out in front, palms down. Bend your hands upward at the wrist, until your hands and forearms make a 90-degree angle. Hold for ten seconds. Relax.

11. HANDS: Extend both arms in front, palms up. Make tight fists and hold tense for ten seconds. Release quickly. Relax.

12. ABDOMEN: Push your stomach muscles out as far as you can. Hold for ten seconds. Release. Now draw in all your stomach muscles, keeping them tight for ten seconds. Release and relax.

13. THIGHS: Press your upper legs together tightly, but don't let the leg areas below the knees touch. Keep that tension for ten seconds, then release quickly. Relax.

14. LOWER LEGS: Sitting on the floor with your legs straight out in front of you, put your feet together and point your toes forward. Hold ten seconds. Now, using your ankles, bend your feet back toward your body as far as possible. Hold for ten seconds. Relax.

15. FEET: Do one foot at a time. First, raise your toes; then bend your whole foot upward, while slowly rotating your ankle away from your other foot. After ten seconds, relax. Next, curl your toes, then your whole foot downward. After ten seconds, relax.

"These exercises may take some practice; you may even be more tense at first," advises Dr. Quentin Regestein, associate professor of psychiatry at Harvard Medical School. "But the more you do them, the greater you'll be controlling your muscle tension, thereby getting on top of stress."

Dr. Lawrence Weitz, clinical psychologist at the Vanderbilt University School of Medicine, adds: "With these exercises, you'll learn how to let go of tension, how to control it."

Everyone can benefit from this program, concludes Dr. Coodley. "You'll switch off the stress alarm button before a ton of stress crushes you."

FROM THE MAUI SUNSET TO THE HULA SLAP— STRESS BEATERS FROM HAWAII

If you have a taste for the exotic, these movements may be just what you're looking for. Think of what your friends will say when they ask you what you're doing and you reply "Why, the Diamond Head Head Roll, of course!"

When you find yourself in a stressful situation, try one or more of the following exercises recommended by University of Hawaii psychiatrist Dr. Danilo Ponce.

1. WALNUT FOOTBALL: While seated, take your shoes off and simply roll a walnut or golf ball under your foot, including the heels and toes, for a minute. Then repeat the exercise with the other foot. "This exercise will relax your foot, leg and calf muscles and provide a sense of general well-being," explains Dr. Ponce.

2. BALI HA'I SIGH: Deeply inhale through your nose, then purse your lips and exhale slowly through your mouth, while letting out an audible sigh. Do the exercise ten times, visualizing your cares blowing away with each breath.

3. DIAMOND HEAD HEAD ROLL: Lower your chin to your chest. Slowly rotate your head up the right shoulder and continue around and down the left shoulder in a complete wide and easy circle. Do this five times. Then straighten up, shrug and wiggle your shoulders. Then do five more head rolls, this time reversing direction.

4. SURFER'S SHOULDER STRETCH: Sit down, close your eyes, relax and slowly rotate your shoulders forward, upward, backward and down. Do four complete rotations one way and four the other way. This exercise is good for a stiff upper back.

5. MAUI SUNSET HEAD REST: Sit down. Let your chin slump to your chest. Close your eyes and picture the most beautiful sunset you've ever seen. Now massage your temples and the corners of your jawbone under each earlobe. Using the tips of all ten

fingers, tap rapidly and gently all over your head and the back of your neck for several minutes. This entire exercise should take between five and ten minutes.

6. TEN FINGER DANCE: Place your arms at your sides and shake your hands vigorously. Bend your elbows, bring your hands up to shoulder height and shake your hands once more. Keeping your elbows bent, make a tight fist with each hand and hold for a minute or two. Now extend your fingers, stretching them into a wide span. Relax and then repeat the entire exercise five times.

7. WATERFALL WRIST ROLL: Sit with your elbows propped on a desk or table. Keeping your hands limp, slowly rotate your wrists—one at a time—in a wide circle. Do this five times in one direction, five times in the other. Then get up and shake your hands, as if you were shaking water from them. Imagine you are shaking off whatever has been causing you to feel stressed. The complete exercise should take around two minutes.

8. PALM TREE PRESS: You rub your palms together briskly till they feel warm. Then quickly cup the palms of your hands over both eyes. With eyes closed, begin to breathe deeply and quietly. Imagine the sound of your breath as a light wind rustling through palm trees. When you feel completely relaxed, you can stop.

9. HULA SLAP: After a bath or shower, use both hands to slap all over your body for a few minutes. This exercise will invigorate you.

10. POLYNESIAN LAGOON DIP: Fill your bathtub with warm water, get in, lean back and relax. Begin breathing very deeply. Each time you exhale, chant the word "a-lo-ha" in as low a tone as you can, dragging out each syllable as long as you can. Repeat at least ten times. This can be the next best thing to a Hawaiian vacation.

The Nutritional Factor

"You are what you eat" has become a cliché in recent years. But it is not as farfetched as many would have you think. If you consider the vast and complex system called "the body," and remember that it is a living, breathing organism which takes in sustenance to help it grow, fight disease and go on living, the question of fuel, or food, can take on new dimensions. If you run or jog or do any sort of rigorous exercise, you probably are more aware of food and its role in helping your body meet the challenge and demands of a race or swim meet or game of tennis. But, even if you are not athletic, you have surely found that, when you don't get enough food, you feel tired or your stomach growls or you develop a headache and get dizzy. Just ask a dieter.

While it is clear to everyone that we all need "a well-rounded diet," what is not clear is just what that means. To many government regulators and medical doctors there is a formula for requirements which encompasses not only the basic food groups, but vitamins and minerals as well. For nutritionists and health food, or natural food, enthusiasts, the role of vitamins and minerals, proteins and amino acids, carbohydrates, fats, bran products and a host of other elements is an ongoing educational project. Many such nutritionists feel that individuals are different and thus have different needs. In addition, they feel that certain diseases, stresses, injuries, etc. all increase each person's needs for varying food and nutritional supplements.

The section that follows is a sample of some of the current thinking and research in this field of nutrition as it relates to stress. It is by no means a complete survey of diet and nutrition and the effects of stress. But it may give you some insight into what are believed to be some of the dietary sources of stress. In addition there is a discussion of a nonprescription, nondrug, pill which has helped some people cope with stress, and some guidelines on the nutritional needs of different age groups. It is always best to discuss questions of diet with your physician, so that he can keep an eye out for any side effects which might arise from a change in diet. Use your common sense, too, and remember that miracle cures which promise to solve all your problems with one tablet, or by eating seaweed, are suspicious to say the very least.

TOO MUCH SUGAR CAN CHANGE YOUR PERSONALITY

Too much sugar in your diet can alter your personality, can make you nervous, irritable, depressed, hostile and even irrational.

"Sugar is a prime producer of stress," says Dr. C. Norman Shealy, a neurosurgeon and leading stress expert. "There are studies that indicate people with too much sugar in the diet have a tendency to become more aggressive, much more easily frustrated, irritable and irrational."

Numerous other experts agree, saying that millions of Americans are suffering simply because they are eating too much sugar. An estimated 20 to 30 percent of the U.S. population—at least 43 million people— suffer some negative effects from too much sugar, according to Dr. Richard Ferman, a Los Angeles psychiatrist who has studied thousands of people who consume too much sugar and experience adverse effects.

"These people can experience nervousness, irritability, anxiety, moodiness and flares of temper," he points out. "They might get to feeling depressed and very down—even to the point of feeling suicidal. They may have irrational fears and phobias and act on these feelings. If they are married or if they have kids, they overreact to situations. They get into fights with their families and may physically abuse them. It jeopardizes their jobs. It can be an extremely destructive pattern."

Dr. Ferman explains that, when you eat sugar, your body tries to get rid of it quickly and often overreacts, so that within a few hours your blood sugar actually falls below normal levels. "As blood sugar drops, people have difficulty concentrating," he explains. "They can't remember, feel mentally dull. Even at its mildest, they find themselves in a negative thinking state—low self-esteem, loss of willpower."

It is estimated that the average American consumes 128 pounds of sugar a year and gets 25 percent of all calories directly from refined sugar.

"The average American is eating thirty-four teaspoons of sugar a day—and we really don't need sugar in the diet," says Dr. U.D. Register, chairman of the nutrition department at Loma Linda University School of Health.

If you must have sugar, Dr. Register recommends a) eating less than ten teaspoons of sugar a day and b) limiting your intake of sugar to mealtimes.

ZAP STRESS WITH VITAMINS AND MINERALS

You can whip stress quickly by using a simple vitamin and mineral plan, say three nutrition experts who created the program. They advise that this simple plan can help an estimated 50 million Americans who suffer stress—and its related problems—due to common vitamin and mineral deficiencies. And it should show results within one week.

Dr. Mary Jane Hungerford, nutrition specialist and codeveloper of the program, says: "This plan can make a tremendous improvement in the well-being of a vast number of Americans. After only a week of taking the vitamins and minerals we recommend, their stress will melt away—meaning they'll become healthier, since stress is the underlying cause of many, many diseases."

Dr. Arthur Furst, a leading researcher and vitamin expert, who also helped devise the plan, agrees that it "can improve the quality of your life. It'll make you feel better and you'll have a better outlook."

On the special program, you simply take *double* the U.S. government's recommended daily allowances (RDAs) of fourteen common vitamins and minerals *for one week*. The following table gives the RDAs.

Vitamin C: 60 milligrams (mg.).
Vitamin B_1: 1.5 mg.
Vitamin B_2: 1.7 mg.
Niacin: 19 mg.
Vitamin B_6: 2.2 mg.
Vitamin B_{12}: .003 mg.
Folic acid: .4 mg.
Biotin: .1 to .2 mg.
Pantothenic acid: 4 to 7 mg.
Iron: 18 mg. for women, 10 mg. for men
Zinc: 15 mg.
Magnesium: 400 mg.
Manganese: 2.5 to 5 mg.
Calcium: 1,000 mg. (1 gram)

You can get most of the fourteen elements in ordinary over-the-counter multivitamin pills, such as Unicap and One-A-Day. Read the label of the product you choose to see which of the fourteen elements it contains. If some elements are missing, or if the multivitamin doesn't contain 100 percent of the RDA for some of them, you'll have to buy individual supplements of those. (Supplements are available in most pharmacies and health food stores.)

For example, if the multivitamin product lacks zinc— one of the plan's fourteen elements—you will need to purchase a separate bottle of zinc supplement.

Likewise, if the multivitamin pill has only a percentage of the RDA of an element—say 10 percent of the needed calcium—you *cannot* just take extra multivitamins to make up the difference, because you'll get too much of the other vitamins and minerals. Again, you'll have to buy a separate calcium supplement.

The fourteen vitamins and minerals listed in the plan act specifically to help stress. You'll find that most multivitamin products contain other elements, such as vitamin E, as well. But don't worry about them, advises Dr. George Briggs, a professor of nutrition and codeveloper of the plan. "They aren't going to hurt you," he says. "In fact, they can aid the elements that are specific against stress."

Although an expert consulted by The NATIONAL ENQUIRER said there is no risk in doubling the RDAs for a week, you should not take more than twice the recommended amounts for more than a week. If your stress has been reduced after one week on the plan, it means that your stress problems were related to a vitamin-mineral deficiency, according to Dr. Furst.

After one week on the plan, cut back your vitamin-mineral intake to the recommended daily allowances, the experts advise. You'll continue to get the same benefits.

Choosing a Vitamin Plan for Your Own Personal Needs

According to Dr. Martin Feldman, a New York nutrition specialist, tens of millions of Americans need more than the U.S. government's recommended daily doses of vitamins, because of their life-style, personal habits and other factors. "This has to be compensated for," he says. "The amounts of vitamins in this plan will do exactly that—and will help those people live a happier, healthier life."

The vitamin plan, created exclusively for The NATIONAL ENQUIRER by top experts, recognizes that different groups of people have different vitamin needs. In every case, your specific tailor-made vitamin program should be taken in addition to a well-balanced diet, which will provide you with the government's minimum daily requirement.

When following this plan, you should, *if you fall into more than one category, take only the highest amount of a vitamin specified in your groups.*

For example, under the plan, senior citizens need one thousand international units of vitamin A and overweight people need five thousand. If you are an overweight senior citizen, then take only five thousand units of vitamin A. *Be sure you do not add the two amounts together.*

Here, according to the experts, are the extra vitamin supplements different groups of people need every day:

CIGARETTE SMOKERS

"Smokers always have a vitamin C level in their blood that is lower than nonsmokers," says Dr. Alton

Ochsner, former chairman of the department of surgery at Tulane University and author of *Smoking and Health*. Therefore, smokers should take at least one thousand milligrams of vitamin C a day, he says. Those who smoke more than a pack of cigarettes a day should take up to two thousand milligrams.

DRINKERS

"Alcohol can literally zap many of your B-complex vitamins," explains Dr. Emanuel Cheraskin, a world-famous nutrition expert. Drinkers—particularly those who consume at least three beers, three glasses of wine or two ounces of liquor a day—should take at least seventy-five milligrams of vitamin B_3 and fifteen to twenty milligrams of vitamin B_6 daily.

WOMEN USING ORAL CONTRACEPTIVES

"Because of their estrogen content, oral contraceptives alter most of the nutrients in the body," Dr. Judy Brown, Ph.D., a University of Minnesota nutritionist, points out. Studies on "the Pill's" effects on women have shown a lack of vitamins B_6 and C in users, adds Dr. Cheraskin. He says that women on the Pill should take fifty to seventy-five milligrams of vitamin B_6 daily and two thousand milligrams of vitamin C.

SENIOR CITIZENS

"If you are over sixty-five, you will need anywhere from five to ten times the government's recommended daily amount of vitamins, with the exception of vitamins A, D and E, which can be dangerous in large amounts," advises Dr. Feldman.

The experts say that both men and women over 65 need sixteen hundred international units of vitamin A, one thousand milligrams of vitamin C, three hundred international units of vitamin D, two hundred to three hundred international units of vitamin E, fifty milligrams of vitamin B_1, fifty milligrams of vitamin B_2, seventy-five milligrams of vitamin B_3, twenty-five to fifty milligrams of vitamin B_6 and one hundred to one hundred fifty micrograms of vitamin B_{12}.

Dr. Feldman warns that senior citizens with a history of heart trouble should check with their doctors before taking vitamin E.

HOUSEWIVES AND OTHER PEOPLE UNDER STRESS

"Stress has a profound effect on your body chemistry —and millions of housewives are attempting to cope with the tremendous pressures of rearing children and taking care of a home," says Dr. Donald Robertson, director of the Southwest Bariatric Nutrition Center in Scottsdale, Arizona.

To combat stress, here's what you need: one thousand or more milligrams of vitamin C, twenty to fifty milligrams of vitamin B_1, twenty to fifty milligrams of vitamin B_2, one hundred to two hundred milligrams of vitamin B_3, twenty-five to fifty milligrams of vitamin B_6 and seventy-five to one hundred micrograms of vitamin B_{12}.

BLUE-COLLAR WORKERS

"A person who performs physical labor on the job tends to use up more B-complex vitamins," advises Dr.

Feldman. "B-complex vitamins burn up very easily during physical activity. If your job involves heavy labor, take half your B vitamins before work and half after work, and you won't use them up on the job. Also, since many blue-collar jobs often require time outside, exposed to the elements, vitamin C can help build up your resistance to infection."

Here is what blue-collar workers need: two thousand milligrams of vitamin C, twenty-five milligrams of vitamin B_1, twenty-five milligrams of vitamin B_2, fifty milligrams of vitamin B_3, fifty milligrams of vitamin B_6 and fifty to seventy micrograms of vitamin B_{12}.

If you work indoors, add four hundred international units of vitamin D to your intake to make up for vitamins you miss out on from not being in the sun, Dr. Robertson suggests.

WHITE-COLLAR WORKERS

"Like those blue-collar workers who spend all their time inside, these people don't get all the vitamin D they need from the sun," says Dr. Robertson. "And, since they don't exercise much, vitamin E is also important to help them better utilize the oxygen that gets to their brain."

White-collar workers need thirty to forty international units of vitamin E, two thousand milligrams of vitamin C, four hundred international units of vitamin D and five thousand international units of vitamin A.

WEEKEND AND OCCASIONAL ATHLETES

"During sports activity, vitamin E is called for to help the cardiovascular system," explains Dr. Feldman.

"And vitamin C helps preserve the connective tissues that are pulled and stretched through exercise."

Occasional athletes should take at least two thousand milligrams of vitamin C, two hundred to four hundred international units of vitamin E, fifty milligrams of vitamins B_1, B_2 and B_3, twenty-five to fifty milligrams of vitamin B_6, and seventy-five micrograms of vitamin B_{12}.

ACTIVE ATHLETES

"Those who engage in sports more than three times a week have special vitamin needs," Dr. Feldman advises. "They tend to eat more protein than they should, and don't get enough complex carbohydrates."

To offset vitamin imbalances, active athletes should have: twenty-five hundred milligrams of vitamin C, fifty milligrams of vitamin B_1, fifty milligrams of vitamin B_2, seventy-five milligrams of vitamin B_3, twenty-five to fifty milligrams of vitamin B_6, seventy-five to ninety micrograms of Vitamin B_{12}, five thousand international units of vitamin A, four hundred international units of vitamin D and two hundred to four hundred international units of vitamin E.

"As in the case of blue-collar workers, try to space out your B-complex vitamins," Dr. Feldman adds. "Take half before your physical activity and half afterward."

ACTIVE TEENAGERS

Most teens are so active, they don't eat proper meals, according to Dr. Robertson. "Bone strength is important to a teenager's good health, and vitamin D is essential to their bones."

A teenager needs: four hundred international units of vitamin D, five hundred to one thousand milligrams of vitamin C, fifteen milligrams of vitamin B_1, fifteen milligrams of vitamin B_2, forty milligrams of vitamin B_3, twenty-five milligrams of vitamin B_6, twenty-five micrograms of vitamin B_{12} and five thousand international units of vitamin A.

OVERWEIGHT PEOPLE

"Believe it or not, overweight people are actually malnourished," reveals Dr. Feldman. "They eat a lot of food, but it's all the wrong kinds. However, the proper combination of vitamin tablets will help make up for what they're not getting in food."

They should include: one thousand milligrams of vitamin C, twenty-five milligrams of vitamin B_1, fifty milligrams of vitamin B_2, fifty milligrams of vitamin B_3, twenty-five millgrams of vitamin B_6, seventy-five micrograms of vitamin B_{12}, five thousand international units of vitamin A, one hundred international units of vitamin D and one hundred to two hundred international units of vitamin E daily.

How Different Foods Affect Your Moods

"Food plays an incredibly important role in the way we feel and act from day to day," says Dr. H.L. Newbold, psychiatrist and author of fourteen books, including *Mega-nutrients for Your Nerves*. "Certain foods make us feel down and depressed, and other foods perk us up and make us feel happy and energetic. Simply by eating the right foods, you can transform yourself from an irritable, depressed grouch into a happy, go-get-'em winner."

Dr. Newbold adds: "Certain foods, such as milk, sugar, sweet foods and grains are 'down' foods. They can help make you depressed, confused and unhappy. Other foods, such as meat and vegetables—the rawer the better—are 'up' foods."

For a happy, upbeat mood, Dr. Newbold recommends the following dietary program:

Eat meats: not processed meat, such as packaged bacon or hot dogs, but real meat, such as beef, pork, liver, lamb, or fowl, such as chicken.

Prepare foods rare, except for pork. The more you cook a piece of meat, the more vitamins are lost.

Eat many different kinds of vegetables, which are a powerhouse of nutrients. Also they contain calcium, which, Dr. Newbold says, "stabilizes the nerve cell membranes and makes the body less excitable."

Use unsaturated fats, such as safflower oil or corn oil on salads. "These oils calm the nerves."

Cut down on sugar and sweet foods or eliminate them altogether. "Sugar can cause depression, nervousness and tension."

Avoid grains and grain products, such as bread and cereals. Grain causes extreme nervousness and depression in many people.

Drink spring water or club soda. The chlorine in tap water can make people irritable, blue and nervous.

Take vitamins. "Be sure to take at least a multivitamin tablet a day to help insure your body is getting all the nutrients it needs to function efficiently and happily."

L-Tryptophan: It Can Perk You Up, Calm You Down and Help You Sleep Like a Baby

L-Tryptophan, which you can buy without a prescription, can effectively combat stress, depression and insomnia. L-Tryptophan is not a drug. It's a totally natural substance, which medical experts say has no harmful side effects, and it is readily available at most health food stores around the country.

"L-Tryptophan is terrific," says world-famous stress expert and neurosurgeon Dr. C. Norman Shealy. "It's safe and at least as effective as any tranquilizer or antidepressant I know. It can help you beat the blues— or even just the blahs. It can help the housewife who's nervous about entertaining her husband's boss, the businessman who's closing a big deal, the student who's cramming for a tough exam. If you're nervous about a job interview, it will relax you."

Best of all, Dr. Shealy adds, L-Tryptophan can replace tranquilizers, sleeping pills and dangerous antidepressant drugs.

In study after study in the United States and Great Britain, L-Tryptophan has been shown repeatedly to eliminate anxiety, mild depression and sleep problems.

Dr. Edith Miller, a neurologist at Maimonides Medical Center in Brooklyn, said that she has been giving L-Tryptophan instead of sedatives and tranquilizers to victims of severe stress. "The results are sensational. I haven't found anything better. It's ideal, because it's a totally harmless substance. For people suffering from stress, it's much better than taking a tranquilizer, because it's not habit-forming.

"Out of an active patient list of eight hundred, I

don't have a single one on sleeping pills. I just give tryptophan. For the elderly (in particular), it's much better than a sleeping pill, because it leaves them clearheaded in the morning."

Psychiatrist Dr. Ivan G. Podobnikar, founder-director of the Ohio Pain and Stress Treatment Center in Columbus, reports that he had been recommending L-Tryptophan to selected patients since he discovered its amazing powers by testing it on himself. "I had undergone four spinal surgeries and suffered from pain and stress," he recalls. "I used L-Tryptophan on a trial basis for several months. It relieved my pain and stress so well that I was able to function with complete efficiency. I became very enthused with it."

Dr. Podobnikar adds that "every person in the U.S. needs L-Tryptophan at one time or another. Everyone has various crises that upset them." The doctor cites the following situations in which the substance would be especially helpful:

1. The healthy housewife who wakes up feeling hung over because of a poor night's sleep—and then gets depressed when she sees all the chores facing her.

2. The athlete who's feeling stress as the "big game" approaches.

3. Youngsters who are upset over schoolwork or teenage problems.

Dr. C. Norman Shealy, founder of the Pain and Health Rehabilitation Center in La Crosse, Wisconsin, says he used L-Tryptophan on more than five hundred severely depressed patients in a three-year period with "excellent" results. He adds that it is almost impossible to overdose on L-Tryptophan. If a huge amount is taken, it is simply disposed of by the body in a natural way.

Apparently, L-Tryptophan occurs naturally in many foods. Some good sources are milk, yogurt, cheese, fish, chicken, meats, beans, peas, eggs and peanuts.

Although it would be helpful to eat more of these tryptophan-rich foods, Dr. Shealy notes that "you cannot get enough L-Tryptophan in the average diet to improve your sleep and relieve stress, anxiety and depression. You would have to take L-Tryptophan supplements to achieve those results."

Most L-Tryptophan sold in this country is imported from Japan. It is extracted from a natural yeast culture and is marketed in 500-milligram (½ gram) or 667-milligram (⅔ gram) tablets or capsules. Dr. Shealy suggests taking one capsule with breakfast. If that isn't adequate, take a second one later in the day. This should combat stress and depression all day and help you get right to sleep that night. It is not necessary to take L-Tryptophan every day—just when you feel special stress.

CHAPTER V

Creating Your Own Antistress Program

SOMETIMES, AFTER READING A BOOK LIKE THIS, IT CAN BE difficult to remember everything you want to try. You can use the Table of Contents, of course, to look up certain sections which you want to refer to again. You can recall certain instances and stories which were right on target for you and your particular stress situations. But normally we don't take the kinds of notes or make the necessary outline which can really be helpful. Sometimes we just want someone to do it for us. If you want an "action agenda" or "action points" that you can follow to begin taking the stress out of your life and to learn to live with the stresses you can't get rid of, this is the chapter you can use as an overall guide.

There are countless magazine articles, newspaper series, TV programs and books on stress—the causes and solutions. They may or may not be related to your specific needs. There are programs devised by the best experts, medical schools, stress clinics and hospitals in the country to relieve stress. They are all valuable on one level or another.

We have examined many excellent plans for dealing

with stress. We have selected four of these plans, deleted the repetitions, reorganized the information and tried to divide the information along approximately the same lines as this book. What we have come up with is an abbreviated, but useful, outline for coping with the stress in your life. It is a starting point only. You alone know your limitations or the limitations imposed on you by your family or job or finances. You have plenty of common sense and you can use it as you look through these guidelines.

Before we begin, here are the four plans we have drawn from: The Mayo Clinic plan as outlined by Dr. Earl T. Carter, professor of preventive medicine at the Mayo Medical School in Rochester, Minnesota, and by Dr. Robert Ivnik, assistant professor of psychology at the medical school; the Baylor College of Medicine stress plan, from the medical college at the Texas Medical Center, Houston; a nine-point program to fight stress from psychologists Robert L. Woolfolk and Frank C. Richardson, coauthors of *Stress, Sanity and Survival;* and a five-step program based on material from the following stress experts: Dr. Hans Selye, director of the International Institute of Stress in Montreal, Dr. Gary Schwartz, Ph.D., professor of psychology at Yale University and professor of psychiatry at Yale School of Medicine, Dr. Barr Taylor, assistant professor of psychiatry at Stanford University and associate director of Stanford's Laboratory for the Study of Behavioral Medicine, Dr. J. Christian Gillin, deputy director of the National Institute of Mental Health's laboratory on clinical psychopharmacology, Dr. C. Norman Shealy, a board-certified neurosurgeon, director of the Pain and Health Rehabilitation Center in La Crosse, Wisconsin, and an internationally known expert on the problems of stress, and Dr. Emanuel Cheraskin, a nationally recognized nutrition expert, professor emeritis at the University of Alabama

Medical School and author of the best-selling book, *Psychodietetics*.

A Self-Help Approach to Living with Stress

1. Stress management begins, says Dr. Seth Silverman at Baylor College of Medicine, with good self-monitoring. Be aware of your feelings, like anger, fatigue, sadness or anxiety. Accepting your feelings frees you to deal with them.

2. Once you are aware of your feelings—your reactions to stressful events—you can learn to control them. Take charge of your response to routine aggravations, advises Dr. Silverman. You can learn to deal with traffic jams, deadlines, financial problems, troubles from your teenage children.

3. Learn to accept what you cannot change. "Try to face things as they are, not as you wish them to be," advises Dr. Robert Ivnik. "If you attempt to change something over which you have no control, you're going to be frustrated. You have to learn to realize the limits of your power and influence, and work within those limits." You can set up and stick to your own family budget, but you cannot influence the national economy or whether the cost of meat will rise in the next year, for example.

4. Make a commitment—write it down—to learn to cope with stress. Put down all the reasons why you feel you need to deal more effectively with stress, and the benefits you look forward to if you succeed. When you get discouraged about the progress you are making, or if you have a setback, reread your statement. Reevalu-

ate the goals you have set for yourself, and remind yourself what is at stake if you give up.

5. Keep a stress diary, or add a special section in the diary you may already keep, for the discussion and identification of sources of stress and your reactions to them. It will help to relieve some of the tension you feel, release some of the emotions you keep bottled up and provide insights into yourself when you reread the section later on. And if you are in a bad situation one day, wondering how you will cope, just flip the pages of your diary back to a year or so before—you may be amazed by what you have survived in the past and be encouraged enough to find the strength to get through bad times again.

6. Talk out your problems. Find someone—a family member, close friend, minister—you can relate to, and lay out your problems on the table. It gives you some relief just to talk things out and it can give you a different point of view about your troubles. Sometimes the simple act of putting your feelings into words can be very therapeutic. Dr. Ivnik adds, "Having the opportunity to review your situation with another person, who might be less partial and biased, might help you keep things in perspective so that you don't overreact."

7. Learn to tolerate and forgive. Psychologists Frank C. Richardson and Robert L. Woolfolk caution that "intolerance of others leads to frustration and anger. An attempt to really understand the way other people feel can make you more accepting of them." You can start by focusing on the good points of the people around you and avoid criticism.

8. Take time to relax. You can often walk away from a source of stress—maybe just for a minute or two in the office—and reduce its influence on you. Or you can literally walk away by taking a stroll outside or sitting alone in a quiet room. It helps to leave your office problems at the office when you can and have fun

during your leisure time. Have some laughs, do things you've never tried before or even try activities you aren't good at—as long as you don't feel you have to win. And try to take time off for vacations; even if you can't go away somewhere, you can enjoy the time away from your daily duties by going on family outings, trying a new restaurant, the movies or other change-of-pace ideas.

9. Set goals and be realistic about them. Whether it is planning household chores for the week ahead or setting up a five-year-plan for buying a new house or car, don't try to do the impossible. If you try to do everything in too little time, you are setting yourself up for disappointment. Make a list of the things you have to do to reach your goal. Decide which are the priority items which have to be done and which are items with an indefinite due date.

Next, tackle the high-priority jobs and, when they are out of the way, set your mind to the lower-priority items. And remember to build in some flexibility. Chores may take longer than you thought, or financial setbacks, such as not getting the raise you expected, can affect your timing. This doesn't mean you have to abandon your goal; you simply have to build in "time cushions" to absorb the shock of setbacks. Also make sure that your list is specific in naming the goal and the steps needed to achieve it. As you finish each step or "mini-goal," cross it off so that you have a sense of movement and accomplishment.

10. Learn relaxation techniques. Through the mental and physical relaxation techniques that are available to you, learn to give your mind a vacation and your body a break from the tension of dealing with stress. Whether it is focusing on one word, a spot on the wall or a pressure point on your forehead, you can learn to relax your mind. And, whether you do head rolls, body stretches, toe wiggling or ankle rotations, you can bring

the same kind of peace to your body through stress-releasing exercises.

11. Take care of your body. Getting a good night's sleep and getting it regularly is one of the building blocks of coping with stress. As sleep expert Dr. J. Christian Gillin suggests, try to stick to a regular schedule for going to bed and getting up; don't nap; be aware that drugs and too much alcohol interfere with your sleeping pattern and that exercise at night can keep you awake; and home remedies like a glass of warm milk, a hot bath or a glass of wine might help you get to sleep.

Remember to eat well. A balanced diet with all the proper nutrients, from protein, to vitamins, minerals, fats, carbohydrates and amino acids, is essential to helping your body cope with the demands of stress.

And, finally, get a regular physical examination. You should know whether you have high blood pressure, adequate hormone production, what your blood sugar level is and a lot of other medical information. If you want to fight stress, you've got to make sure your body is up to the battle.

Conclusion

IF MISERY LOVES COMPANY, THEN BOY COULD WE BE IN love. Just think of all the people you know who complain about the pressures of life, and keep multiplying by ten. It doesn't seem to get any easier either. Experts say our lives are getting more and more complicated with each passing decade. But the news isn't all bad. If you're married, you are healthier and suffer less stress than single people, according to a University of Pittsburgh study. That's because you have someone "to confide in," says psychiatrist Dr. Neil Pauker. "You can go home and pour your heart out to a spouse about your troubles at work."

But, if you and your spouse both work, you may be headed for some unexpected trouble—especially if you are a man. Two psychiatrists, Dr. Irving Tracer, with the Michael Reese Hospital and Medical Center in Chicago, and Dr. Sidney Lecker, at Mount Sinai Hospital in New York, agree that, while working women are under greater pressure from their jobs and families, they handle it better than men. They also have fewer heart attacks, ulcers and high blood pressure problems than men. One reason, says Dr. Tracer, that women cope better is they are "more open about their feelings" and can release tension through very frank and open discussions. Men tend to bottle up their emotions and are afraid to cry.

On the other hand, men have it over women when it comes to changing values and sex roles. New York University psychologist Dr. George Serban conducted a study of over one thousand men and women and found that, by 81.8 percent to 53.8 percent, women are more upset by sexual permissiveness than men. And 81.4 percent of working married women say their jobs interfere with their marriage, while only 56.4 percent of the men feel the same way.

One of the most surprising surveys, however, is the one about who suffers more stress, bosses or secretaries. A government survey of stressful occupations found that secretaries rank second on the list. Lack of authority, lack of opportunity for upward mobility in the company and boredom with the job are some reasons cited by University of Maryland professor Dale Masi. And furthermore, bosses tend to unload their own tensions on their secretaries.

All that these examples demonstrate is that nobody avoids stress. And life's complications aren't just small aggravations, they are hurting us—our mental and physical health are suffering. But what we have learned in this book is that there are answers. We can reduce the ill effects of living with stress. We can change our attitudes and behavior and learn to control how we deal with stress. We can even begin to take advantage of stress by learning from it and using it as a signal that something is wrong. We can stop trying to be supermen and super-women and concentrate on doing as much as we can, as well as we can. We can talk to our loved ones and friends, and listen as well. We can take control of our lives. No, we are never going to be able to control the ravages of nature gone wild, or the contrariness of an economic slump. But we can learn to live with stress and live pretty darn good lives while we are doing it.

The choice is really all ours.

The next time you want to punch out the gas station attendant, just stop and think "Is this how I want to live my life? Do I really want to go from one confrontation to another?" The next evening you are sitting around waiting for your husband to get home from work, and thinking of all the rotten things you want to say to him to make him pay for ruining the dinner, ask yourself "Do I want to ditch this guy or am I going to figure out, with him, how to deal with last-minute business meetings that wreck our evenings?" And the next time you're ready to chew your secretary out for typing a letter the wrong way, take a minute to remember whether you might have dictated it wrong.

Misery probably doesn't really like company; it probably just wants an end to misery. If you think about it—so do we all.